D0953103

HIV/AIDS in Young Adult Novels

An Annotated Bibliography

Melissa Gross
Annette Y. Goldsmith
Debi Carruth

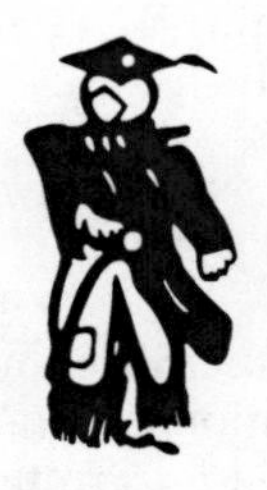

THE SCARECROW PRESS, INC.
Lanham • Toronto • Plymouth, UK
2010

Published by Scarecrow Press, Inc.
A wholly owned subsidiary of The Rowman & Littlefield Publishing Group, Inc.
4501 Forbes Boulevard, Suite 200, Lanham, Maryland 20706
http://www.scarecrowpress.com

Estover Road, Plymouth PL6 7PY, United Kingdom

British Library Cataloguing in Publication Information Available

Library of Congress Cataloging-in-Publication Data

Gross, Melissa.
HIV/AIDS in young adult novels : an annotated bibliography / Melissa Gross, Annette Y. Goldsmith, Debi Carruth.
p. cm.
Includes bibliographical references and index.
ISBN 978-0-8108-7443-5 (alk. paper) — ISBN 978-0-8108-7444-2 (ebook)
1. Children's stories, American—Bibliography. 2. Young adult fiction, American—Bibliography. 3. AIDS (Disease)—Juvenile fiction—Bibliography. 4. AIDS (Disease)—Fiction—Bibliography. 5. HIV infections—Juvenile fiction—Bibliography. 6. HIV infections—Fiction—Bibliography. 7. Children's stories, American—Stories, plots, etc. 8. Young adult fiction, American—Stories, plots, etc. 9. Teenagers—Books and reading—United States. I. Goldsmith, Annette Y. II. Carruth, Debi. III. Title.
Z1232.G76 2010
[PS374.A39]
016.813'54093561—dc22 2010020714

∞™ The paper used in this publication meets the minimum requirements of American National Standard for Information Sciences—Permanence of Paper for Printed Library Materials, ANSI/NISO Z39.48-1992.

Printed in the United States of America.

Contents

Foreword

Ten-year-old Natasha showed me the teddy bear she was knitting in her after-school craft club. "It's for orphans in Africa," she said. "Are they AIDS orphans?" I asked. "I don't know," she answered. "What's AIDS?"

Natasha's parents are progressive and liberal in their child-rearing approach. Both her mother and father have talked with her about sex. Yet neither they nor her teachers nor the adult running the craft club had thought to tell her about AIDS. Natasha is an avid reader and may encounter some of the novels discussed in this guide over the next few years. Reading *Earthshine* or *Night Kites* might have been her first informational encounter with a health issue of devastating global consequences.

The authors of *HIV/AIDS in Young Adult Novels: An Annotated Bibliography* make a convincing case for the need to inform young people who are living in the age of the AIDS epidemic about the facts of the disease. They also present a passionate argument for fiction as a means of transmitting social norms, values, and contextualized information about a topic as potentially controversial or sensational as HIV/AIDS. They are also brutally honest about the limitations of the current published body of work. For every novel that is both accurate and well written, there are others that present misinformation in didactic or pedestrian prose.

This, then, is the added value that Melissa Gross, Annette Goldsmith, and Debi Carruth have provided in this guide to teen novels about HIV/AIDS. They have made an exhaustive search for fiction on this topic, looking beyond the usual trade books published in the United States to small presses and novels published in English far beyond our borders. They have used a rigorous content analysis methodology to quantify relevant elements of plot and character, HIV/AIDS content, and literary quality. The well-written, thorough annotations in the bibliographical section are further aids to understanding the usefulness and overall quality of the books in question.

Many adults who may believe that teens should be informed about HIV/AIDS may still feel insecure about their own level of knowledge or about good strategies for communicating facts. This guide will help to alleviate those insecurities and hopefully contribute to a generation of teens better informed and better able to make personal and political choices involving HIV/AIDS.

Virginia A. Walter
Professor Emerita
University of California, Los Angeles

Introduction: What Do Young Adult Novels Have to Say about HIV/AIDS?

The HIV/AIDS epidemic has now been with us for more than twenty-five years. Although great strides have been made in terms of treatment, there is still no vaccine or cure; therefore, prevention measures, especially those concerned with the young adult population, have mainly focused on education concerning how HIV is transmitted and how individuals can keep themselves safe from HIV infection. It has been reported that a full 88 percent of U.S. high school students have received education about HIV/AIDS in school.[1] However, other reports give evidence that young people are still very much in jeopardy. Many lack the information they need to keep themselves safe as well as to respond empathetically to those who have the virus. Many are also still misled into thinking that HIV/AIDS is someone else's problem, not something that is likely to touch their own lives. This thinking began early in the epidemic with the perception that HIV/AIDS was a disease that preyed only on certain groups, such as gay men and drug users. The idea of HIV/AIDS as a problem for someone else continues today, with the perception that the virus primarily occurs in developing countries, too far away to affect adolescent life in the United States.

Another reason to be concerned about what young people know about HIV/AIDS is that even when education is provided, information about the facts of the disease is often insufficient to change behaviors. As Albert Bandura notes, information alone

> has not slimmed the obese, eradicated cigarette smoking . . . or made a substantial dent in nutritional patterns that create high risk of cardiovascular disease in those who need to change most. It certainly will not make the sexually active celibate and impel intravenous drug users to renounce drugs, which are the two major modes of HIV transmission.[2]

In addition to facts, young adults need skills that will allow them to manage relationships, make sound decisions, and have the self-esteem necessary to believe that they can control their behaviors and influence their social environment. Fiction is a natural vehicle for modeling these skills and their development within the context of social landscapes that are relevant to young people.

A content analysis of media coverage of HIV/AIDS from 1981 through 2002 demonstrated that public opinion no longer views HIV/AIDS as an urgent health problem in the United States, and subgroups known to be disproportionately affected by the epidemic receive little attention from the news media.[3] The young adult population is one of these subgroups in which the incidence of newly diagnosed infections continues to grow quietly. The Henry J. Kaiser Family Foundation reports that half of new HIV infections occur in people under the age of twenty-five, and that in 2002, more than half (51 percent) of infections in thirteen- to nineteen-year-olds were found in young women.[4] Infection in young women is mainly due to heterosexual transmission, another indication that AIDS is no longer a problem only for isolated subgroups of the population.

In addition to numbers of new infections, the Centers for Disease Control and Prevention (CDC) reports that the number of youth ages thirteen to twenty-four living with AIDS increased 42 percent between 2000 and 2004.[5] Furthermore, although the risk of vertical transmission has decreased, children infected with HIV at birth or by blood transfusion are now living longer and are part of the adolescent population.[6] Also, due to improved treatments, more youth are living with family members who have HIV/AIDS. For infected youth and those touched directly by the presence of HIV/AIDS in their lives, the stigma still associated with the disease is a very real concern. The fear of being stigmatized can affect the ability of HIV-positive individuals to trust in others and may keep them from disclosing their status even as they form intimate relationships.[7]

At the same time research reports that among young adults concern about contracting HIV is minimal and misconceptions about how the disease is transmitted persist, including beliefs that the disease can be contracted through kissing, sharing a drinking glass, or from a toilet seat.[8] A recent survey of young adults reports that 87 percent of respondents "do not believe that they are at risk for HIV infection."[9] The CDC, in highlighting the risks youth face, especially minority youth, states, "Continual HIV prevention outreach and education efforts, including programs on abstinence and on delaying the initiation of sex, are required as new generations replace the generations that benefited from earlier prevention strategies."[10]

Librarians, teachers, health professionals, parents, and other adults interested in youth continue to have an important role to play in helping young people understand the HIV/AIDS epidemic. This includes providing information about the facts of transmission, as well as the facts related to the social, emotional, and societal implications of the epidemic. Young adult fiction is particularly well suited to dealing with the multidimensional nature of this need, as it has the potential to provide facts and debunk myths, provide models for how to handle difficult social situations, and arouse critical thinking and empathy in readers.

Unfortunately, it is difficult to identify fiction that contains subject matter about HIV/AIDS, as these books are seldom catalogued for this content, nor is this content consistently revealed in published reviews. This makes it difficult to suggest titles to young people or interested adults, as well as to know which books contain useful information for young people, for use in the classroom, or to promote discussion in other information providing contexts.

The overriding question that framed this project from its inception is, If all that young adult readers knew about HIV/AIDS was the result of reading fiction, what would they know about the epidemic, how the disease is transmitted, and the level of risk HIV/AIDS poses for them personally? John Goldthwaite says that, "every book teaches. It teaches the world it portrays and imprints us with a sense of how we are to respond to that world."[11] This perspective guides the interpretations of the HIV/AIDS information these books contain. We also maintain the point of view that books are social artifacts in which are embedded adult messages for young people.[12] The specific questions that guide this work include the following:

- Which characters have HIV/AIDS in these novels?
- What is their relationship to the protagonist?
- How did they contract the disease?
- What fears, if any, does the protagonist have about contracting HIV/AIDS?
- Is HIV/AIDS depicted as a condition that can be controlled?
- What is the fate of HIV/AIDS characters?

The books considered in this project are written for young adults ages eleven to nineteen, contain a protagonist in this age range, are written in or translated into English, are fiction, and contain at least one character who is HIV positive or who has AIDS. The first book of young adult fiction published that meets this criteria is *Night Kites* by M. E. Kerr, published in 1986. This is one of four books that earned Kerr the American Library Association's Margaret A. Edwards Award in 1993. When Kerr wrote this book, she was so sure that a cure for AIDS would soon be found that she left in current day music references that she otherwise would have edited from her story.[13] Unfortunately Kerr, like many, was mistaken about this, and in the absence of a cure, HIV/AIDS remains a very real concern.

As of 2008, there have been ninety-three young adult novels identified that meet the criteria of this study. We have read and analyzed each for the information it conveys about living in the age of the AIDS epidemic. We sought to determine the merits of each book individually, as well as the entire set as a body of literature. The discussion of the content of these books, used with the annotated bibliography, will facilitate the identification of these novels and provide an assessment of their content for librarians, teachers, and other interested adults, as well as young adults themselves. It is hoped that this will be an invaluable resource for choosing, collecting, evaluating, and using these works as a component of strategies to educate readers about HIV/AIDS.

Toward this end, this book is arranged in two parts. Part I: HIV/AIDS Content in Young Adult Novels presents various analyses of the HIV/AIDS information provided in this subset of young adult literature. Part II: Annotated Bibliography, 1981–2008 provides a complete listing of all ninety-three young adult novels identified by the authors and includes full citations and an annotation for each entry. In addition, each entry is labeled in terms of the accuracy of the HIV/AIDS information it provides, the centrality of HIV/AIDS to the story told, and an assessment of the literary quality of the work.

Part I is made up of five chapters, each focused on a different aspect of the novels contained in the bibliography. Chapter 1, "HIV/AIDS Novels for Young Adults," discusses the methods used to find the books discussed here as well as how the content of these works was analyzed. The remaining chapters in this section provide in-depth discussions of the questions used to frame this inquiry.

Chapter 2, "Who Has HIV/AIDS and How Did They Get It?," is concerned with who the HIV/AIDS characters in these novels are and how these characters contracted the disease. The age, gender, and the HIV/AIDS characters' relationship to the protagonist are all considered in terms of how they frame the reader's view of HIV/AIDS. Such questions as the following are discussed: Are young adults depicted as being at risk or is HIV/AIDS primarily seen as an adult problem? Is HIV/AIDS a disease that strikes strangers or is it primarily a problem for people outside of the United States? To what extent are HIV/AIDS characters in these books people that the protagonists know and care about? Are any of these young adult protagonists themselves infected? This chapter also addresses how HIV/AIDS characters become infected and the extent to which the reasons given represent real risk factors for young adults. For instance, reliance on explanations of tainted blood and blood products or vertical transmission provides a different picture of risk than do characters infected via intravenous drug use or unprotected sex.

Chapter 3, "What Are We Afraid Of? Protagonist Views of Risk," assesses the extent to which young adult protagonists voice fears related to HIV/AIDS and the kinds of fears they have. This chapter includes a discussion of what constitutes reasonable and unreasonable fears, what worries protagonists have for their own welfare, and what anxieties they experience related to the welfare of others. We also consider whether the type of fears discussed in these novels has changed over time.

Chapter 4, "How Controllable Is HIV/AIDS?," considers whether HIV/AIDS is presented as a chronic or a terminal illness. In the early days of the epidemic, infection with the HIV virus was thought to be a death sentence. Today, people in the United States are living longer thanks to the availability of new drugs, but does this mean that being infected is not worth worrying about? This chapter discusses the views of protagonists concerning how controllable HIV/AIDS is, what kind of control is discussed (drugs, nutrition, positive thinking, etc.), and other issues, such as access to medical care. This analysis also considers whether the depiction of the disease as controllable or uncontrollable has changed in these novels during the time period considered. This chapter also considers another aspect of the risk posed by the AIDS epidemic, related to messages about how controllable the disease is, and that is whether HIV/AIDS characters in these books survive or die. It also explores the extent to which the fate of HIV/AIDS characters is experienced as living with HIV or dying of AIDS and whether the attitudes toward the fate of people infected with HIV have changed as new treatments have been developed.

Chapter 5, "Young Adult Novels with HIV/AIDS Content as a Body of Literature," summarizes the points made throughout the book concerning how young adult novels deal with various dimensions of the AIDS epidemic. It provides a generalized discussion of the strengths and weaknesses of this body of young adult literature and answers the question, If all that young adult readers knew about HIV/AIDS was the result of reading fiction, what would they know about the epidemic, how the disease is transmitted, and the level of risk HIV/AIDS poses for them personally?

NOTES

1. Centers for Disease Control and Prevention (CDC), "HIV/AIDS among Youth," 2006. Available at www.cdc.gov/hiv/resources/factsheets/PDF/youth.pdf (19 November 2009).

2. Albert Bandura, "A Social Cognitive Approach to the Exercise of Control over AIDS Infection," in *Adolescents and AIDS: A Generation*

in Jeopardy, ed. Ralph J. DiClemente (Newbury Park, CA: Sage Publications, 1992), 89.

3. M. Brodie, E. Hamel, L. A. Brady, J. Kates, and D. E. Altman, "AIDS at 21: Media Coverage of the HIV Epidemic, 1981–2002," Kaiser Family Foundation, 2004. Available at www.kff.org/kaiserpolls/AIDS at21.cfm (18 November 2009).

4. Kaiser Family Foundation, "National Survey of Teens on HIV/AIDS," 2000. Available at www.kff.org/youthhivstds/upload/National-Survey-of-Teens-on-HIV-AIDS.pdf (18 November 2009).

5. Centers for Disease Control and Prevention, "HIV/AIDS among Youth," 2006.

6. Geri R. Donenberg and Maryland Pao, "Youths and HIV/AIDS: Psychiatry's Role in a Changing Epidemic," *Journal of the American Academy of Child and Adolescent Psychiatry* 44, no. 8 (2005): 728–47.

7. Lori S. Wiener, Haven B. Battles, and Lauren V. Wood, "A Longitudinal Study of Adolescents with Perinatally or Transfusion Acquired HIV Infection: Sexual Knowledge, Risk Reduction, Self-Efficacy, and Sexual Behavior," *AIDS Behavior* 11, no. 3 (2007): 471–78. José Ricardo de Carvalho Mesquita Ayres, Vera Paiva, Ivan França Jr., Neide Gravato, Regina Lacerda, Marinella Della Negra, Heloisa Helena de Sousa Marques, Eliana Galano, Pilar Lecussan, Aluísio Cotrim Segurado, and Mariliza Henrique Silva, "Vulnerability, Human Rights, and Comprehensive Health Care Needs of Young People Living with HIV/AIDS," *American Journal of Public Health* 96, no. 6 (2006): 1001–6.

8. Brodie et al., "AIDS at 21," 2004. Kaiser Family Foundation, "National Survey of Teens on HIV/AIDS," 2000.

9. Long Island Association for AIDS Care, Inc. (LIAAC), "Youth and HIV Statistics," 2005. Available at www.heart-intl.net/HEART/120606/Youth&HIV.htm (19 November 2009), para. 7.

10. Centers for Disease Control and Prevention, "HIV/AIDS among Youth," 2006, para. 1.

11. John Goldthwaite, *The Natural History of Make-Believe: A Guide to the Principal Works of Britain, Europe, and America*. (New York: Oxford University Press, 1996), p. 75.

12. Anne Scott MacLeod, "An End to Innocence: The Transformation of Childhood in Twentieth-Century Children's Literature," in *Opening Texts: Psychoanalysis and the Culture of the Child*, eds. Joseph H. Smith and William Kerrigan (Baltimore: John Hopkins University Press, 1985). Virginia A. Walter, *War and Peace Literature for Children and Young Adults: A Resource Guide to Significant Issues* (Phoenix, AZ: Oryx, 1993).

13. Alleen Pace Nilsen, "M. E. Kerr," in *Writers for Young Adults*, Vol. 3, ed. Ted Hipple (New York: Charles Scribner's Sons, 1997).

1

HIV/AIDS CONTENT IN YOUNG ADULT NOVELS

1

HIV/AIDS Novels for Young Adults

Perhaps it goes without saying that in order to study the HIV/AIDS content of young adult novels it is necessary to be able to identify the books that include information about HIV/AIDS in the story; however, there are several difficulties that immediately present themselves in relation to finding these books. One issue that must be clarified is identifying who the assumed audience for these works is, or put another way, making clear how *young adult* is defined. Another problem is the need to set parameters for what constitutes a young adult novel, particularly since what young adults read can run the gamut of everything from children's to adult books. When these two concepts are clarified, the problem then becomes how to find young adult books that have the required HIV/AIDS content so that they can be read, coded, and analyzed.

The following is a discussion of how the terms *young adult* and *young adult literature* are defined for this study and a description of the process used to identify books to be included in this study.

WHO ARE YOUNG ADULTS?

There are several names people use to refer to young adults, such as *teenagers* or *adolescents*; however, as much at home as we are with these terms, the idea that people experience a special developmental stage between childhood and adulthood is a relatively new idea. At the beginning of the twentieth century people went directly from childhood to adulthood as they entered apprenticeships or otherwise became wage earners or married. The period of adolescence as a distinct phase between childhood and adulthood was first described by psychologist G. Stanley Hall in 1904, with the publication of *Adolescence: Its Psychology and Its Relations to Physiology, Anthropology, Sociology, Sex, Crime, Religion, and Education*.[1] Hall saw adolescence as a tumultuous period but also one which if properly handled could have a positive impact on the evolution of humanity.

Since the emergence of the idea of adolescence as a distinct period of development, the time at which people enter adulthood has been shortened and lengthened depending on the needs of society.[2] Such societal issues as the number of jobs available, the enactment of child labor laws, the institution of mandatory school attendance, and the need for military personnel have all affected the point at which individuals have been considered adults. For example, during periods when jobs have been scarce, young people have been encouraged to stay in school longer. In contrast, in times of war, many young people have been deemed adult enough to join the military. Recently, however, in Western culture the period known as adolescence has increased in length. The need for a college education to be competitive in the job market has become more important, and many young people are choosing to postpone marriage and parenthood until they establish their careers.

This change has led another psychologist, Jeffrey Jensen Arnett, to propose that human development now includes another stage between adolescence and adulthood, which he calls "emerging adulthood."[3] He classifies emerging adulthood as taking place in the eighteen- to twenty-nine-year-old year range. He describes this period as one in which people are deeply involved in self-exploration concerning love and work issues.

As Hall notes, young adulthood also has a biological aspect to it; therefore, one approach to defining the concept of young adulthood is to tie it to physical development and the onset of puberty. Of course, the age range within which individuals reach puberty is quite wide, starting for some as early as ten years of age and for others not beginning until age sixteen. These two factors, biology and social issues, make it difficult to nail down an exact age range during which an individual will be considered a young adult. The Young Adult Services Association (YALSA), a division of the American Library Association, focuses on services to those in the twelve- to eighteen-year-old year range; however, YALSA acknowledges the limitations to service in adopting this age range by pointing out that, "Adolescence begins in biology and ends in culture."[4]

For this study, young adults are defined as eleven- to nineteen-year-olds. This age range captures young people likely to be in middle school and high school and strives in this way to cover this population and its special concerns without including others who are more likely to be representative of children or emerging adults.

WHAT ARE YOUNG ADULT BOOKS?

Just as the definition of young adults as a group is in many ways a constructed one that varies based on biology and societal influences, conceptualizing young adult literature and what young adults read varies according to the maturity of the reader. This has led several writers to define this body of literature as anything young adults read. While today there are books that are written and published specifically for young adults, young adults have long been known to choose reading from books published for adults and also, at times, to return to literature meant for children.

Michael Cart reports that many books we now think of as young adult novels were initially published for adults.[5] Examples include works by Louisa May Alcott, Charles Dickens, Jules Verne, and Mark Twain. The ALEX Award, which has been administered by YALSA since 1998, acknowledges the ongoing importance of adult books for young adult readers. The ALEX Award honors ten adult books each year that have special appeal to young adults.

While it was not written specifically for young adults, the 1942 publication of Maureen Daly's *Seventeenth Summer* is often used to mark the beginning of young adult publishing.[6] However, the first novel published specifically for young adults, *Sue Barton, Student Nurse*, by Helen Boylston, arrived on the scene six years earlier.[7] Early young adult literature was dominated by stories of romance, adventure, career, and sports. These books have a general reputation as superficial stories and did little to advance the idea that young adult books could be thought of as "literature"; however, over time the character of young adult novels has evolved. In the late 1960s, S. E. Hinton's *The Outsiders* marked a sea change in which young adult books began to tackle serious developmental and social issues and move toward a more realistic depiction of life. The "problem novel" has become a mainstay of young adult literature. Such serious topics as sexual abuse, substance abuse, abandonment, and neglect are integrated into much of young adult literature, as are the breakdown of the traditional family unit, difference in socioeconomic backgrounds, race relations, and the inclusion of gay and lesbian characters. While other genres, such as romance and fantasy, have continued to be produced and have an important place in fiction meant for young adults, contemporary realism is at the heart of young adult literature in terms of library and classroom markets.[8]

For this study, the common wisdom that young adults prefer to read about characters like themselves led to the decision to include books that have a protagonist in the age range we have used to define young adults, that is, eleven to nineteen years old. Novels specifically written for young adults are emphasized, but works of fiction written for adults or children, in which the main character is a young adult, were also considered to be part of what young adults might reasonably read. All genres of fiction are acceptable in this study. Short stories are excluded. Works sought were limited to those published in English. Books published before 1981 were not considered, as 1981 marks the date of the first reports of immune system disorders among gay men and injecting drug users.

WHAT IS A YOUNG ADULT NOVEL ABOUT HIV/AIDS?

To isolate young adult novels that have HIV/AIDS content, it was important to find a definition that captured some information about HIV/AIDS in a way that would ensure that the resulting set of books could be both identified and located. The main problem behind this issue is the limitation of identifying books based on subject headings and the small number of finding aids, for example, subject bibliographies, available on this topic.

There are many books that mention HIV/AIDS in passing, perhaps to say that something about it was brought up at school or as a piece of gossip, or even to lament the existence of the disease. Some books of this type include Jenny Davis's *Sex Education*,[9] *When She Hollers* by Cynthia Voigt,[10] and Francesca Lia Block's *Witch Baby*.[11] There are also books that make reference to the fear of contracting HIV/AIDS as a passing remark. Examples of these include Barbara Wersba's *Just Be Gorgeous*,[12] Mary Dowling Hahn's *The Wind Blows Backward*,[13] and Pete Hautman's *Sweetblood*.[14] In the case of David Levithan's novel of the near future, *Wide Awake*,[15] HIV/AIDS is briefly noted as a disease of the past.

Including books at the level of anything that mentions HIV/AIDS, however, did not make sense in that it would be very difficult, if not impossible, to ensure that each one of these books could be identified and located. To define a body of young adult works of fiction with HIV content in which there could be more certainty that the whole population could be accounted for, a more discoverable definition was needed. The solution was to isolate young adult novels that included at least one character who is HIV positive or who has AIDS, regardless of how central to the plot this character might be.

While this definition provides a more discoverable body of literature, one downside, which only became apparent at the end of the study, is that it excludes books that are about HIV/AIDS but that do not include a character who is HIV positive or who has AIDS. An example of this kind of book is Terry Trueman's *7 Days at the Hot Corner*,[16] which tells the story of a young man waiting for the results of his HIV test. This novel has a lot to say about HIV/AIDS and fear and is a book that readers interested in the topic of HIV/AIDS will want to know about.

Patricia McCormick's novel *Sold*[17] is an example of a different type of book excluded from the study, one in which there may well be HIV/AIDS information, but it is not manifest. In this novel about a Nepalese girl sold to a brothel, there are characters with sexually transmitted diseases, but since the words *HIV* and *AIDS* never appear in the text, it is impossible to identify them as being HIV positive.

IDENTIFYING TITLES

For this study, works of fiction were sought that have the following characteristics:

- Have a main character in the young adult age range (eleven to nineteen)
- Have at least one character who is either HIV positive or who has AIDS
- Are written in English
- Were published between 1981 and 2008

However, identifying this body of books requires much diligence as subject headings, book summaries, book annotations, book jacket information, and reviews often do not identify HIV/AIDS content in a novel, especially when HIV/AIDS is not a major theme. To help overcome this limitation, in addition to subject headings that explicitly identify HIV/AIDS content, related subject headings such as those indicating content related to drug use/abuse, sexuality, sexual abuse, challenged materials, death and dying, nontraditional families, gay and lesbian content, homelessness, runaways, and so forth, were also used to try to identify HIV/AIDS content.

Between 1987 and 1999, some finding aids were available in library literature that concentrated on HIV/AIDS resources for youth. These took the form of short bibliographies published mainly in such review journals as the *Wilson Library Bulletin*, *School Library Journal*, *Booklist*, and so forth. During this period there were also several articles published in the library literature that addressed the need for library services to respond to the information needs of young people regarding HIV/AIDS. All of these articles were utilized and provided a foothold into this literature related to early publishing efforts in this area.

In addition to these finding aids, resources used to identify books that met our definition included the following:

- Standard bibliographies
- Specialized bibliographies
- Standard book review outlets (*Horn Book*, *Booklist*, *VOYA*, etc.)
- SIECUS reports

- Catalog searches (World CAT, Library of Congress, etc.)
- Database searches (Children's Literature Comprehensive Database, Database of Award-Winning Children's Literature, TeachingBooks.net, ATN Book Lists, Books in Print, etc.)
- Online bookseller searches (Amazon.com, Barnes and Noble, etc.)
- Postings to professional Listservs (CCBC-Net, Child_Lit, etc.)
- Web searches for individual titles and book lists
- Searches of professional association websites (ALA, IRA, IFLA, etc.)
- Searches of proprietary databases (Library Literature, JSTOR, Education Full Text, etc.)
- Queries to publishers and writers
- Queries to colleagues and friends

A list of published resources used is provided at the end of this chapter. The search for titles was iterative and took place over several years as we read and coded the books we identified. In some cases we noted that it can take years for a title to appear in finding aids, and so it is possible that a few books may have been missed, particularly if published within the last few years.

DATA ANALYSIS

All of the titles identified and discussed in this book have been read, coded, and analyzed by all three of the authors. The analysis was guided by the following research questions:

- Which characters have HIV/AIDS in these novels?
- What is their relationship to the protagonist?
- How did they contract the disease?
- What fears, if any, does the protagonist have about contracting HIV/AIDS?
- What is the fate of HIV/AIDS characters?

For each of these questions a coding sheet was developed (see Appendix F) on which were recorded pertinent content and page numbers where the content is located. The questions were designed to capture manifest content to minimize the need to interpret meaning and therefore the subjectivity of the coding.

However, at times interpretation was required. For example, coding the age of characters is easy when the text manifestly says what the character's age is: "Bite me. He's only twenty-five."[18] But when a specific character's age (or other needed coding) is not overtly stated, sometimes it can be derived from the context. For example, it is often clear that an uncle, teacher, or teacher's husband is an adult by virtue of his or her position and/or relationship to the protagonist and is coded as such. When clues to a character's age are provided, these were used to substantiate the coding. When there was insufficient information to construct a coding item, it was coded as "unknown."

All books were read and coded independently by each of the study's authors. The individual coding sheets were then compared to ensure the quality of the coding and to ensure that all coders agreed about what the text said. In almost all instances, the initial coding of the books reflected a high level of agreement between all three coders. When coding did not agree, the coding was discussed until consensus was reached and great care was taken to ensure the consistency of the coding approach across all coding when interpretation was required. For example, in novels set in Africa the most common way that HIV is spread is through heterosexual sex.[19] Therefore, in the absence of other content about how infected characters in Africa acquired the virus, such as intravenous drug use or homosexuality, an assumption of heterosexual transmission was held. Likewise, infants infected with HIV were assumed to have contracted the disease from their mothers. After all the books were coded and the coding was compared and discussed, the data was entered into SPSS, statistical software designed for use in the social sciences, to facilitate statistical analysis.

In addition to coding the books for content related to the research questions, a full annotated bibliography of all of the books was developed as a finding aid for readers and others interested in identifying, reading, and using these books. Each entry is headed by a complete bibliographic citation that includes the author's name, title of the book, place of publication, publisher's name, and ISBN for the edition of the book that was used in the coding. Where information about a previous edition of the work is available, this has been included in the citation. Entries are in alphabetical order by the author's last name. The following is a sample citation:

> **VAN DIJK, LUTZ.** *Stronger Than the Storm.* Translated from German by Karin Chubb. Cape Town: Maskew Miller Longman Pty., Ltd., 2000. [Originally published as *Township-Blues* by Elefanten Press Verlag GmbH in 2000.] ISBN 0-636-04476-9 (paperback)

Each entry in the bibliography is rated in terms of the accuracy of the HIV/AIDS content it provides, the centrality of HIV/AIDS to the story, and its literary quality. These ratings are provided to give the reader a sense of the book at a glance. Four rating levels for HIV/AIDS content are defined. These include accurate, accurate but some implausible content, accurate but dated, and inaccurate. Three levels of centrality are used to specify the role HIV/AIDS has in the story. These are central to plot, a subplot, and mentioned in passing. Five levels of literary quality are used to assess the books. These include excellent, very good, good, passable, and poor. All assessments are based on the consensus opinions of the study's authors. These ratings are displayed immediately after the full citation as follows:

> *HIV/AIDS Content Scale:* Accurate
> *HIV/AIDS Role in Story Scale:* Central to plot
> *Literary Quality Scale:* Very good

An annotation describing and evaluating the title follows these ratings. Each annotation considers both the narrative content and the HIV/AIDS content provided in the story. Indexes are provided that list works by the centrality of HIV/AIDS to the story to further expedite access to books of interest for readers.

NOTES

1. G. Stanley Hall, *Adolescence: Its Psychology and Its Relations to Physiology, Anthropology, Sociology, Sex, Crime, Religion, and Education* (New York: Appleton, 1904).

2. Miriam Braverman, *Youth, Society, and the Public Library* (Chicago: American Library Association, 1979).

3. Jeffrey Jensen Arnett, *Emerging Adulthood: The Winding Road from Late Teens through the Twenties* (New York: Oxford University Press, 2004).

4. Young Adult Services Association, *Directions for Library Services to Young Adults*, 2nd ed. (Chicago: American Library Association, 1993).

5. Michael Cart, *From Romance to Realism: Fifty Years of Growth and Change in Young Adult Literature* (New York: HarperCollins Publishers, 1996).

6. Cart, *From Romance to Realism*, 1996.

7. Helen Boylston, *Sue Barton, Student Nurse* (New York: Signet, 1984). Original published in 1936.

8. Pam B. Cole, *Young Adult Literature in the 21st Century* (New York: McGraw Hill, 2009).

9. Jenny Davis, *Sex Education* (New York: Orchard, 1988).

10. Cynthia Voigt, *When She Hollers* (New York: Scholastic, 1994).

11. Francesca Lia Block, *Witch Baby* (New York: HarperCollins, 1991).

12. Barbara Wersba, *Just Be Gorgeous* (New York: Harper & Row, 1988).

13. Mary Dowling Hahn, *The Wind Blows Backward* (New York: Clarion, 1993).

14. Pete Hautman, *Sweetblood* (New York: Simon Pulse, 2004).

15. David Levithan, *Wide Awake* (New York: Knopf, 2006).

16. Terry Trueman, *7 Days at the Hot Corner* (New York: HarperTeen, 2007)

17. Patricia McCormick, *Sold* (New York: Hyperion, 2006).

18. Dakota Chase, *Changing Jamie* (Round Rock, TX: Prizm Books/Torquere Press, 2008).

19. AVERT, "Women, HIV, and AIDS," 2009. Available at www.avert.org/women-hiv-aids.htm (9 October 2009).

RESOURCES USED TO IDENTIFY BOOKS

Baffour-Awuah, Margaret. "Fiction as a Tool to Fight the HIV/AIDS Battle." World Library and Information Congress: 70th IFLA General Conference and Council, August 22–27, 2004, Buenos Aires, Argentina. Available at: http://ifla.queenslibrary.org/IV/ifla70/papers/082e-Baffour-Awuah.pdf.

Blumenreich, Megan, and Marjorie Siegel. "Innocent Victims, Fighter Cells, and White Uncles: A Discourse Analysis of Children's Books about AIDS." *Children's Literature in Education* 37, no. 1 (March 2006): 81–110.

Bradburn, Frances Bryant. "Informing Youth about AIDS: Responsible Resources." *Wilson Library Bulletin* 67 (January 1993): 43–46.

Bradburn, Frances Bryant. "Middle Readers' Right to Read." *Wilson Library Bulletin* 65 (March 1988): 37–43.

Bradburn, Frances Bryant. "Sex, Lies, and Young Readers at Risk." *Wilson Library Bulletin* 65 (October 1990): 34–38.

Campbell, Patricia J. "The Young Adult Perplex: Sources on AIDS." *Wilson Library Bulletin* 62 (September 1987): 71–72+.

Cart, Michael. "Carte Blanche: Silence Still Equals Death." *Booklist* 91, no. 14 (1995): 1,319.

Cart, Michael. *From Romance to Realism: Fifty Years of Growth and Change in Young Adult Literature.* New York: HarperCollins Publishers, 1996.

Cart, Michael, and Christine A. Jenkins. *The Heart Has Its Reasons: Young Adult Literature with Gay/Lesbian/Queer Content, 1969–2004.* Lanham, MD: Scarecrow Press, 2006.

Carter, Betty. *Best Books for Young Adults: The Selections, the History, the Romance.* Chicago: American Library Association, 1994.

Cole, Pam E. *Young Adult Literature in the 21st Century.* New York: McGraw Hill Higher Education, 2009.

Darby, Mary A., and Miki Pryne. *Hearing All the Voices: Multicultural Books for Adolescents.* Lanham, MD: Scarecrow Press, 2002.

Day, Frances A. *Lesbian and Gay Voices: An Annotated Bibliography and Guide to Literature for Children and Young Adults.* Westport, CT: Greenwood Press, 2000.

Deveny, Mary Alice. "Teens in Transition: A Workshop on Teen Sexuality and AIDS for Youth-Serving Professionals." *Voice of Youth Advocates* 16 (October 1993): 209–10+.

"Does AIDS Hurt? A Reading List for Children, Young Readers, and Teens." *Unabashed Librarian* 91 (1994): 17–19.

Eaglen, Audrey. "AIDS to Understanding." *School Library Journal* 36 (August 1990): 105.

Elderton, William E. *Not Just a Schoolgirl Crush: An Annotated Book List of Teenage Novels on the Issues of Being Lesbian.* Available at www.dunedinmethodist.org.nz/mtke/lesb.htm.

Fichtelberg, Susan. *Encountering Enchantment: A Guide to Speculative Fiction for Teens.* Westport, CT: Libraries Unlimited, 2007.

Fitch, Don D. "AIDS: What Every School Media Specialist Needs to Know." *Indiana Media Journal* 10 (1988): 11–15.

Fonseca, Anthony J., and June M. Pulliam. *Hooked on Horror: A Guide to Reading Interests in Horror Fiction.* Westport, CT: Libraries Unlimited, 1999.

Fonseca, Anthony J., and June M. Pulliam. *Hooked on Horror: A Guide to Reading Interests in Horror Fiction*, 2nd ed. Westport, CT: Libraries Unlimited, 2002.

Freebury, Dorie. "Young Adult Fiction about AIDS: An Annotated Bibliography." *Voice of Youth Advocates* 18 (October 1995): 209–10.

Garden, Nancy. "Dick and Jane Grow Up Gay: The Importance of (Gay) Young Adult Fiction." *Lambda Book Report* 3, no. 7 (1992): 7–10.

Gillespie, John T., ed. *Best Books for Young Teen Readers, Grades 7 to 10*. New Providence, NJ: R. R. Bowker, 2000.

Gillespie, John T., and Catherine Barr. *Best Books for High School Readers: Grades 9–12*. Westport, CT: Libraries Unlimited, 2004.

Gillespie, John T., and Catherine Barr. *Best Books for High School Readers: Grades 9–12*. Supplement to the First Edition. Westport, CT: Libraries Unlimited, 2006.

Hautman, Pete. *Sweetblood*. New York: Simon Pulse, 2004.

Helbig, Aletha, and Agnes R. Perkins. *Dictionary of American Young Adult Fiction, 1997–2001: Books of Recognized Merit*. Westport, CT: Greenwood Press, 2004.

Herald, Diana T. *Teen Genreflecting: A Guide to Reading Interests*. Westport, CT: Libraries Unlimited, 1997.

Herald, Diana T. *Teen Genreflecting: A Guide to Reading Interests*, 2nd ed. Westport, CT: Libraries Unlimited, 2003.

Hofacket, Jean. "Intensive Care: Materials on AIDS and HIV." *Library Journal* 118 (January 1993): 65–68.

International Association of School Librarianship (IASL). *AIDS and HIV and School Libraries: Fiction Books for Young People*. 2003 Annual Conference, July 7–11, 2003, Durban, South Africa. Available at http://iasl-slo.org/conference2003-aidsfiction.html.

Jones, Patrick, Patricia Taylor, and Kirsten Edwards. *A Core Collection for Young Adults*. New York: Neal-Schuman Publishers, 2003.

Kaywell, Joan F. *Adolescents at Risk: A Guide to Fiction and Nonfiction for Young Adults, Parents, and Professionals*. Westport, CT: Greenwood Press, 1993.

Koelling, Holly, ed. *Best Books for Young Adults*, 3rd ed. Chicago: Young Adult Library Services Association, 2007.

Lukenbill, W. Bernard. *AIDS and HIV Programs and Services for Libraries*. Englewood, CO: Libraries Unlimited, 1994.

Lukenbill, W. Bernard. "Providing HIV-AIDS Information for Youth in Libraries: A Community Psychology and Social Learning Approach." *Journal of Youth Services in Libraries* 9 (Fall 1995): 55–67.

Mandell, Phyllis Levy. "AIDS Spelled Out on Film: A Videography." *School Library Journal* 40 (May 1994): 54–59.

Middle and Junior High School Library Catalog. New York: Wilson, 1995–2008.

Mueller, Julie M., and Virginia Moschetta. "AIDS Information Sources." *School Library Journal* 34 (September 1987): 126–30.

Ngoshi, Hazel T., and Juliet S. Pasi. "Mediating HIV/AIDS Strategies in Children's Literature in Zimbabwe." *Children's Literature in Education* 38, no. 4 (2007): 243–51.

Prater, Mary A., and Nancy M. Sileo. "Using Juvenile Literature about HIV/AIDS." *Teaching Exceptional Children* 33, no. 6 (2001): 34–45.

Prosenjak, Nancy, Laura Sullivan, and Diane Hartman. "HIV/AIDS: What You Don't Know Can Kill You." In *Using Literature to Help Troubled Teenagers Cope with Health Issues*, ed. Cynthia A. Bowman (pp. 217–41). Westport, CT: Greenwood Press, 2000.

Salvadori, T. R. "AIDS Materials for Children and Young Adults." *New Jersey Libraries* 25 (1992): 6–7.

Sanchez, Alex. *Rainbow Boys and Rainbow High: Novels about Love and Friendship for Teens and Adults*. Available at http://alexsanchez.com/gay_teen_books.htm.

Senior High School Library Catalog. New York: H. W. Wilson Co., 1981–2006.

Silvey, Anita. *500 Great Books for Teens*. Boston: Houghton Mifflin, 2006.

Strobach, Stasis. "The Face of AIDS in Realistic Fiction." *School Libraries Activities Monthly* (February 1999): 12–14.

Tillapaugh, Meg. "AIDS: A Problem for Today's YA Problem Novel." *School Library Journal* 39 (May 1993): 22–25.

Walter, Virginia A., and Melissa Gross. *HIV/AIDS Information for Children: A Guide to Issues and Resources*. New York: H. W. Wilson Company, 1996.

York, Sherry. *Children's and Young Adults Literature by Latino Writers: A Guide for Librarians, Teachers, Parents, and Students*. Worthington, OH: Linworth Publications, 2002.

Zola, Jim. "What Our Children Are Dying to Know: AIDS Information Dissemination and the Library." *North Carolina Libraries* 51 (1993): 142–44.

2

Who Has HIV/AIDS and How Did They Get It?

"Most kids just think AIDS is something that could never happen to them."

—Angela Elwell Hunt, *A Dream to Cherish*[1]

Which characters get HIV/AIDS? How is the disease transmitted? These two research questions are primary to understanding what young adult novels with an HIV-positive character communicate about the risk of transmission of HIV/AIDS and who should be concerned about these risks. Who actually has the disease matters, as does the manner in which it is contracted. By comparing the information in the books to what science has learned about HIV/AIDS, it is possible to see how closely the novels reflect the facts.

This study considers who has HIV/AIDS in these novels in three ways: (1) the relationship of the character with HIV/AIDS to the protagonist, (2) the gender of the infected individual, and (3) the infected individual's age. It is assumed that the closer the protagonist's ties to the character with HIV/AIDS, the greater the likelihood that that person's illness will be meaningful to the protagonist. The health of an immediate family member, for example, will engage the protagonist more directly than, say, that of a minor character with whom the protagonist does not interact. Gender is included as a variable because it is now understood that the disease strikes both males and females. Age is noteworthy because it is assumed that the protagonist will notice and be affected by the existence of HIV-positive characters relatively close in age to himself or herself. So, too, is it assumed that young adult readers will be more drawn to characters in their age group.

In addition to well-defined characters, there are other less distinct indications of people with HIV/AIDS. For example, some of the books reference statistics or prevalence rates as well as individuals. This study sought to capture those who, while not part of the main action of the story, help form the backdrop or context in which the plot takes place. For example, the presence of HIV/AIDS hotlines or specially designated hospital wards assumes the existence of people who require those services without necessarily identifying specific individuals. Indications of characters with HIV/AIDS that were not distinct enough to be counted as individuals were coded as "uncountables." Even though these characters could not be counted, it was important to capture their presence. The overall number of characters with HIV/AIDS in each book was of interest because it indicates the prevalence of the disease; the presence of "uncountables" in the literary landscape accomplishes a similar goal.

There are only three ways in which someone can contract HIV/AIDS: (1) through unprotected sex, (2) vertical transmission (from infected mother to child in utero or through breastfeeding), and (3) contaminated blood. Since the blood supply was made safe in 1985, it has been very rare for hemophiliacs or others requiring blood transfusions to contract the disease. Infection via contaminated blood is more likely to occur now through the sharing of needles or syringes to inject intravenous drugs or, sometimes in a health care setting, through needlesticks.[2]

CODING WHO HAS HIV/AIDS

Different categories of relationships were coded on the assumption that the HIV/AIDS content would be more meaningful to the protagonist if someone close to him or her had contracted the disease. The possible relationships ranged from the closest (self) to no relationship at all. Family, friends, and others who play a role in the protagonist's life, whether these are relationships of necessity or choice, are defined below.

Coding decisions were made from the point of view of the protagonist. If a relationship changed through the course of the narrative, the closest relationship between the character with HIV/AIDS and the protagonist was coded. For example, in *The Heaven Shop*, Jeremiah is a friend of the protagonist's grandmother and so is coded as "family friend."[3] Jeremiah also becomes the protagonist's sister's love interest, but the coding reflects the closer relationship of "family friend." If there are multiple protagonists, the closest relationship among them and the HIV/AIDS character was coded. An example of this may be found in *The Mayday Rampage*, where there are two protagonists, Jess and Molly, only one of whom, Molly, is HIV positive.[4] Therefore Molly was coded as "self." When choices had to be made, it was to err on the side of closeness in the coding, on the assumption that the closest relationships to the protagonists were the most important ones to track in the novels.

Relationship

Self

The closest possible relationship to the character with HIV/AIDS is when the protagonist himself or herself has the disease. Examples include feisty high school journalist Molly in *The Mayday Rampage*;[5] Amanda, *At Risk*'s prize-winning gymnast;[6] and Alex, the new kid in town in *Fade to Black*.[7]

Immediate Family Member

This category includes parents and siblings of the protagonist, broadly defined to include stepparents and foster children. For example, in *Chanda's Secrets*, there is Chanda's stepfather, Jonas,[8] and in *The Case of the Missing Melody*, Jessica's foster sister, baby Melody.[9] The books include a variety of parental circumstances. Some parents live with their offspring, as in *The Heaven Shop*, where Binti's father is the head of the household.[10] There are also estranged relatives like Holden's mother in *Dream Water*, who comes home only when she is ill.[11] In *Singing the Dogstar Blues*, Joss's mother never reveals the identity of Joss's father, and Joss grows up essentially fatherless.[12] Joss does not learn that Daniel Sunawa-Harrod is her father until after his death. Although their connection is unknown for most of the narrative, Sunawa-Harrod was coded as "immediate family member" because of his biological relationship to Joss.

An older sibling often contracts the disease, as happens to Erick's brother, Pete, in *Night Kites*,[13] and Lacy's brother, Jack, in *My Brother Has AIDS*.[14] *Far and Beyon'* describes a situation in which two brothers, Thabo and Pule, have died of HIV/AIDS by the time the narrative begins; their siblings, protagonists Mosa and Stan, must carry on.[15] Older sisters with HIV/AIDS are also in evidence, as in *Playing with Fire*, where Sophia's sister Rosa contracts the disease,[16] and in *What You Don't Know Can Kill You*, in which Debra's sister Ellen discovers she is HIV positive.[17] There are also younger siblings, usually babies, such as Chanda's sister Sara, whose funeral Chanda must arrange.[18]

Extended Family Member

Aunts, uncles, cousins, and grandparents qualify for this category. The degree of family separation from the protagonist does not indicate the depth of the emotional bond. In *I Never Got to Say Good-Bye*, Uncle Mark is more like a brother to Traci than an uncle.[19] Uncle Wolfgang has been estranged from Hand's family in *Oasis*, although not from Hand himself.[20] In *The Beat Goes On*, Leyla's cousin, Emma, the character with HIV/AIDS, is also her close friend.[21]

Teacher

Adults who take on the role of a teacher are included here, which means bona fide teachers such as Jess's favorite teacher, Mr. Goodban, in *The Mayday Rampage*,[22] and Sarah's art teacher, Mr. Hill, in *Rumors and Whispers*.[23] Jason's principal, Mr. Carr, in *Unfinished Dreams*, is also coded as a teacher-like figure.[24]

Friend

This category includes friends with whom the protagonist has a strong personal attachment, and it is distinct from love interests. For example, *The Silent Killer*'s protagonist Natasha and her close friend Jasmine swear that they will tell one another everything; their friendship is tested when Jasmine starts secretly dating an older boy and contracts HIV/AIDS.[25] In *When Love Comes to Town*, Neil shows his attachment to his new friend Eddie, a transvestite who goes by the name Daphne, by visiting him at his home when Eddie is dying of AIDS.[26] Protagonist Barbara and her little sister Livvy literally run into a clown on a bicycle in *Touch of the Clown*, thus forming a strong friendship with HIV-positive Cosmo, who helps the girls cope with their dysfunctional home life.[27] In books 2 through 5 of the Laurel Shadrach Series, *Totally Free*,[28] *Equally Yoked*,[29] *Absolutely Worthy*,[30] and *Finally Sure*,[31] Laurel prides herself as being a good Christian but finds maintaining her friendship with the irritating Brittany, who happens to be HIV positive, a definite cross to bear.

Love Interest

Protagonists' love interests include girlfriends like Alex's lover, Leigh, in *Fade to Black*;[32] Elaine's former fling, Dean, in *Red Hair Three*;[33] and a partner in a committed relationship, such as Robin's partner Stone, in *Robin's Diary*.[34] HIV-positive Jeremy was coded as Nelson's love interest in *Rainbow Boys*,[35] *Rainbow High*,[36] and *Rainbow Road*.[37] Although Nelson is one of three protagonists in this trilogy, Jeremy is closest to Nelson, so it is this close relationship that was captured instead of the more distant "friend's love interest," which is Jeremy's relationship to Kyle and Jason.

Family Friend

Characters in this category are akin to friends who may seem like family but, strictly speaking, are not. Often they are neighbors. In *Chanda's Secrets*, Chanda's family friend, Emmanuel, is the son of Chanda's interfering neighbor, Mrs. Tafa.[38] Likewise, in *Far and Beyon'*, Cecilia and her little daughter, Bibi, are longtime neighbors and friends of Stan and Mosa's family.[39]

Teacher's Family/Friend

There are some characters with HIV/AIDS who the protagonist knows through a teacher. In *Be Still My Heart*, Allie meets Mr.

Adams through his wife, who is one of her favorite teachers.[40] Jess is shocked at the deterioration in the health of Vic, his teacher's partner, when he visits the couple at home in *The Mayday Rampage*.[41] In *My Brother Has AIDS*, Lacy's swimming coach (the equivalent of a teacher) tells her about his HIV-positive brother.[42]

Classmate

A classmate is someone to whom the protagonist has a limited personal attachment. He or she belongs to the same peer group and may be in the same class or just the same school. No classmates were coded. There are certainly classmates in the books, but they are not coded that way because the coding scheme works from the protagonist's point of view. For example, Alex and Clinton are both protagonists but also classmates in *Fade to Black*.[43] As the HIV-positive character, Alex is coded as "self." Since Clinton is not HIV positive, he would not be coded as "classmate" in relation to Alex. Similarly, in *Baby Alicia Is Dying*, Desi is the protagonist.[44] Desi's sister Val has a classmate at college who is HIV positive, but since Val is not a protagonist, her classmate is coded only in relationship to Desi as "no direct relationship."

Friend's Family/Friend

This is a person who is part of a friend's family or a friend of that friend. Quite a few parents of friends are in this category, including Mr. and Mrs. Macholo, Chanda's friend Esther's parents, from *Chanda's Secrets*;[45] the mothers of Leyla's friends, Shula and Ellie, in her HIV/AIDS support group in *The Beat Goes On*;[46] Thina's friend Thabang's mother, in *Stronger Than the Storm*;[47] and the mother of Maybe's friend, 2Moro, in *Can't Get There from Here*.[48]

In books that are part of a series, characters can take on different relationships based on who is the protagonist in a given book. Baby Melody is Jessica's foster sister and is coded as "immediate family" in *The Case of the Missing Melody*.[49] However, in the sequel, *The Mystery of the Poison Pen*, there is a different protagonist, Alysha, and Jessica is the protagonist's friend.[50] Hence Melody is coded there as "friend's family."

An example of a friend of a friend may be found in *Diving for the Moon*, in which Josh asks his gay adult friend at the lake, Elliot, if he has ever had any friends with AIDS: "'Not now. I did have one.' Elliot paused. 'But he died.'"[51]

Friend's Love Interest

This category consists of a person with whom the protagonist's friend is (or was) romantically involved. For example, in *Until Whatever*, Karen's friend Connie has an unnamed former boyfriend who, she later learns, was HIV positive.[52] Similarly, in *Purity Reigns*, Laurel learns that her friend, Brittany, was involved with Justin, who has since been diagnosed with HIV: "Justin and Brittany were quite an item for awhile, and he was the first guy she had ever been intimate with."[53]

Immediate Family Member's Love Interest

This is a person with whom the protagonist's parent or sibling is romantically involved. Unbeknownst to Liam in *The Eagle Kite*, his father is having an affair with a young man named Geoff.[54] In *What You Don't Know Can Kill You*, Debra's older sister, Ellen, has a boyfriend, Jack.[55] Lacy's brother in *My Brother Has AIDS* had a partner, Lincoln, who died of AIDS.[56]

Extended Family Member's Love Interest

This category includes the love interest of an aunt, uncle, cousin, or grandparent. Examples are 2Moro's aunt's boyfriend, who is briefly mentioned in *Can't Get There from Here*,[57] and Uncle Wolfgang's partner, Bernard, in *Oasis*.[58]

Fictional Characters

Though strictly speaking, all of the characters are fictional, two of the books contain characters who are fictional within the narrative. In *The Heaven Shop*, there are several characters in a radio play designed to promote HIV/AIDS awareness,[59] and the main character in the musical *Rent* is referenced in *Fade to Black*.[60]

Other Miscellaneous Characters

These are people the protagonist is aware of but may or may not know personally. Anne hears about but never meets her caregiver's son in *Sixteen and Dying*,[61] while *University Hospital: Heart Trauma* medical students Zoey and Tristan see pediatric patient, Bishop Wilson, regularly.[62]

No Direct Relationship

These are characters with whom the protagonist is unlikely to interact. They include people glimpsed and forgotten, such as a homeless person in *I Was a Teenage Fairy*[63] and a few nameless street people in *Random Acts of Senseless Violence*.[64] Such celebrities as Magic Johnson in *The Mayday Rampage*,[65] Rock Hudson in *Until Whatever*,[66] and Arthur Ashe in *What about Anna?*[67] are also mentioned. Although the protagonist will have heard of the celebrity, there is little chance that they will ever meet. Some characters are present merely to infect another character and further the plot, including the rapist in *Now That I've Found You*[68] and the person with whom Arien shared needles in *A Dream to Cherish*.[69] There are adults and some young adults in hospitals, clinics, and support groups. Examples include the people at the hospital in *The Heaven Shop*,[70] the patients in the AIDS ward in *Rumors and Whispers*,[71] and members of an HIV/AIDS support group in *I Never Got to Say Good-Bye*.[72]

Individuals memorialized in the AIDS quilt and associated ceremonies also have no direct relationship to the protagonist. In *Tommy Stands Alone*, visitors "pay tribute to the people whose faces and names were on the panels of the quilt."[73] In *Zach at Risk*, Zach reads aloud a page of names in commemoration: "Donald Wallace, Scott Finch, Melissa DeSoto, James Lee Dare."[74]

Statistics and "Uncountables"

Some of the books provide statistics to show the extent of the illness. For example, in *Robin's Diary* Robin does some research and discovers that there have been "441,528 cases of AIDS diagnosed and reported since 1981."[75] This information was captured, but the actual figures were not included in the total number of characters calculated for each title. Rather, they were considered evidence of the prevalence of the disease. There were also indications of the pandemic that did not mention individuals with HIV/AIDS but made it clear that they existed. These indications were dubbed "uncountables." Passages noting an AIDS hotline, people in an AIDS ward, or graveyards full of AIDS victims were recorded because they attest to the extent of the pandemic and help provide the backdrop against which the narrative is told.

Gender

There are three categories: (1) male, (2) female, and (3) unknown. The gender of characters was considered unknown if insufficient information was available to make this assessment. For example, in *Notes from a Spinning Planet: Papua New Guinea*, Maddie and her journalist aunt hear about a "couple of AIDS cases" in the village but have no idea if they are male or female.[76] No categories for intersex, transgender, and so forth, characters were used because no such characters with HIV/AIDS were found in this set of novels.

Age

Age was coded in one of the following mutually exclusive categories: nonviable pregnancy or miscarriage, young child (birth–age 4), school-age child (ages 5–10), young adult (ages 11–19), emerging adult (ages 20–25), adult (ages 26–64), and senior (ages 65+). If it could be deduced from manifest evidence in the text that the age spanned two of those ranges, the following combined categories were used: school-age child/young adult (ages 5–19), young adult/emerging adult (ages 11–25), emerging adult/adult (ages 20–64), and adult/senior (ages 26–65+). However, if the possible age spanned more than two ranges, or if there was no information at all, it was coded as "unknown."

CODING HOW HIV/AIDS IS TRANSMITTED

Since HIV/AIDS can only be transmitted through unprotected sex, vertical transmission, and infected blood or blood products, these three categories were the basis of the coding. There were separate categories for heterosexual sex, homosexual sex, vertical transmission, intravenous drug use, and infected blood/blood products. The "not known" category was used when no information about the cause of infection was available. Since the coding process relied on manifest text, the coders decided not to bring in outside knowledge to supplement the text. For example, it is common knowledge that Ryan White contracted HIV/AIDS through infected blood products, but if the cause was not mentioned in the text, it was coded as "not known." "Multiple risk factors" was chosen when more than one category of the potential source of infection applied. The addition of an "other" category made the coding scheme comprehensive.

Heterosexual Sex

This category describes sex between a man and a woman as the cause of the HIV infection. In the books that treat the HIV/AIDS pandemic in Sub-Saharan Africa, if no other information is given it was assumed that heterosexual sex was the cause. Statistically, this is how the majority of HIV transmission occurs in the region.[77]

Homosexual Sex

This category describes sex between two people of the same gender as the cause of the HIV infection. In the absence of other manifest risk factors, this was the cause ascribed to HIV infection among characters described as homosexual.

Vertical Transmission

Not all babies born of infected mothers will develop the disease themselves; this category included only those children or youth identified as having been born with HIV/AIDS. For example, in *Notes from a Spinning Planet: Papua New Guinea*, "two of Pilada's children" are said to be infected.[78] Likewise, Gabe and Chloe in *Soul Love* reveal to Jenna that they were both born HIV positive.[79]

Intravenous Drug Use

This category includes "hard" drugs like heroin but also the steroids many athletes resort to to bulk up their muscles, which is what high school athlete Monk does in *Get It While It's Hot. Or Not*: "'It was steroids,' Elaine whispers in Bio. . . . 'That's how

Monk got it,' she whispers. 'He shared a needle with some other muscle-head.'"[80] The infection itself comes from needle-sharing.

Blood/Blood Products

Contaminated blood transfusions as well as blood products for hemophiliacs fall into this category. A blood transfusion during a life-saving operation after a near-fatal car accident is the explanation given for Amanda's condition in *At Risk*,[81] Anne's in *Sixteen and Dying*,[82] and Mark's in *I Never Got to Say Good-Bye*.[83] Josh, in *Diving for the Moon*, is a hemophiliac who contracts HIV/AIDS through contaminated blood products.[84] Accidental needlesticks were also coded here: Medical staff members are infected in *Rumors and Whispers*.[85] In *Insatiable*, Jessica's father, a nurse, "contracted the disease in the course of his work."[86] There is also the case of a policeman attacked with a used needle while on duty, as reported in *The Mayday Rampage*.[87]

Not Known

If absolutely no information is offered as to the cause of transmission and the context does not imply the cause (e.g., unprotected heterosexual sex in one of the novels set in Africa), it was coded as "not known." This is the case in *Life Magic*, when Uncle Joe comes to live at Crystal's house and the reader is offered no inkling as to how he contracted the disease.[88]

In cases where characters are very minor, have no direct relationship to the protagonist, or are vaguely described, risk factors cannot be assumed. For example, in *I Was a Teenage Fairy*, there is insufficient information provided to determine the cause of this man's infection: "A homeless man in the gutter with his head in his hands and a sign that read HAVE AIDS PLEASE HELP propped up against his deteriorating shins."[89] Similarly, in *The Eagle Kite*, the source of infection is a mystery: "a man looking like a scarecrow came to haunt the church steps"[90] holding a sign that read "'I'M HUNGRY I GOT AIDS PLEASE.'"[91]

Multiple Risk Factors

This category was used if there is more than one plausible reason for the cause of transmission. For example, in *Born Blue*,

Janie's Mama Linda may have contracted HIV/AIDS through drugs or multiple sex partners; the reason is not definitive.[92] Lee, in *Ran Van: Magic Nation*, is a former drug addict and is in a homosexual relationship.[93] There are intimations of yet more risk factors in his case: "'It wasn't hard,' Lee said. 'I was in all the categories.'"[94] Rita, Precious's friend in *Push*, also could have contracted HIV/AIDS in any number of ways, as she recounts in her autobiographical assignment: "Foster care, rape, drugs, prostitution, HIV, jail, rehab."[95]

Other

Since the set of novels includes fantasy and science fiction, "other" causes were indeed possible. In *Singing the Dogstar Blues*, for example, the surgical implant of a mechanism to boost one's intelligence brings with it a "one in five chance of crushing your immune system" and the concomitant risk of AIDS infection.[96]

FINDINGS: WHO HAS HIV/AIDS?

As described above, this research question was analyzed in terms of the protagonist's relationship to the character with HIV/AIDS and that character's gender and age. The analysis includes individuals as well as "uncountables," those indications of the presence of people with HIV/AIDS (i.e., hotlines and dedicated clinics). "Uncountables" may also be described in terms of prevalence statistics. Findings are presented in the next section.

Relationship

Figure 2.1 displays the relationship of the HIV/AIDS character to the protagonist in terms of frequency. Nine (2.4 percent) of the 376 characters with HIV/AIDS are themselves young adult protagonists. There are 34 (9 percent) immediate family members with HIV/AIDS and 13 (3.5 percent) extended family members. Four teachers (1.1 percent) figure among those characters who are infected, as do 32 (8.5 percent) friends of the protagonist. Ten (2.7 percent) love interests and 10 (2.7 percent) family friends have HIV/AIDS. There are 5 (1.3 percent) instances of a teacher's fam-

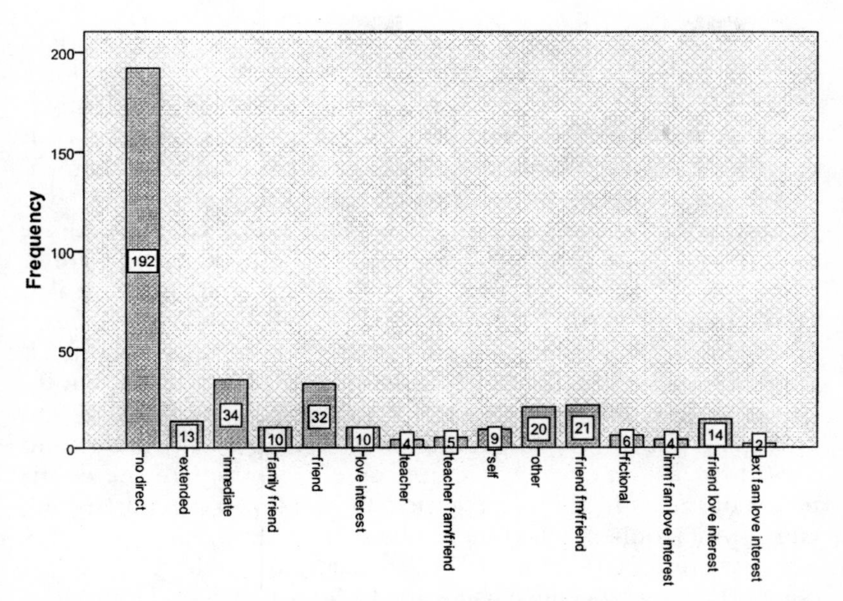

Figure 2.1. Relationship of Characters with HIV/AIDS to the Protagonist

ily or friend who is infected. No classmates were coded. Twenty-one (5.6 percent) characters were coded as a friend's family or friend and 14 (3.7 percent) as a friend's love interest. Four (1.1 percent) characters are the love interest of an immediate family member and 2 (0.5 percent) the love interest of an extended family member. Six (1.6 percent) fictional characters were recorded. There are 20 (5.3 percent) other miscellaneous characters. Just more than half of the characters with HIV/AIDS, 192 (51.1 percent), have no direct relationship to the protagonist.

Two hundred and forty seven separate quotes documenting the presence of "uncountables" were coded in 52 (56 percent) of the 93 books.

Gender

Of the 376 characters with HIV/AIDS, more than half (218 or 58 percent) are male, while 112 (29.8 percent) are female. For 46 (12.2 percent) of the characters, there is insufficient evidence to identify gender, so these characters were coded as "unknown."

In most relationship categories there are more males than females. Indeed, the four teachers, five teacher's family members or friends, four love interests of an immediate family member, fourteen friend's love interests, and two love interests of an extended family member are all males. In several other categories males also outnumber females. Of the 192 characters with no direct relationship to the protagonist, 105 (54.7 percent) are males, 43 (22.4 percent) are females, and 44 (22.9 percent) are of unknown gender. The "other" miscellaneous characters are also predominantly male: 17 (85 percent) are males and 3 (15 percent) are females. This pattern is also true of friends, of whom 18 (56.3 percent) are males and 14 (43.8 percent) are females; family friends with 6 (60 percent) males and 4 (40 percent) females; and protagonist love interest, numbering 7 (70 percent) males and 3 (30 percent) females. There are some exceptions to the dominance of males in these categories. Of the 9 (2.4 percent) young adult protagonists who themselves have HIV/AIDS, 7 (77.8 percent) are female while 2 (22.2 percent) are male. The 21 (5.6 percent) characters coded as a friend's family or friend consist of 13 (61.9 percent) females and 8 (38.1 percent) males.

The gender split is equitable in two categories. Among immediate family members who are infected, there are 16 (47.1 percent) males, 16 (47.1 percent) females, and two (5.9 percent) unknown. The fictional characters are also evenly divided, with 3 (50 percent) males and 3 (50 percent) females. In the category of extended family members with HIV/AIDS, there are almost the same number: 7 (53.8 percent) males and 6 (46.2 percent) females.

Age

Table 2.1 presents the characters with HIV/AIDS by age. In order of frequency, adult is the largest category, with 146 (38.8 percent) cases, followed by "unknown," with 69 (18.4 percent) cases. There are 54 (14.4 percent) young adults and 33 (8.8 percent) emerging adults. The combined category of emerging adult/adult comes next, comprising 28 (7.4 percent) cases. In addition, there are 18 (4.8 percent) young children, 14 (3.7 percent) in the combined category of young adult/emerging adult, and 9 (2.4 percent) school-age children. The remaining three categories include only

Table 2.1. Age of Characters with HIV/AIDS

	Frequency	*Percent*
Miscarriage	2	0.5
Young child	18	4.8
School-age child	9	2.4
Young adult	54	14.4
Emerging adult	33	8.8
Adult	146	38.8
School-age/young adult	2	0.5
Young/emerging adult	14	3.7
Emerging adult/adult	28	7.4
Adult/senior	1	0.3
Unknown	69	18.4
Total	376	100.0

1 (0.3 percent) or 2 (0.5 percent) cases. It is noteworthy that there are no seniors and only 1 (0.3 percent) adult/senior.

FINDINGS: HOW HIV/AIDS IS TRANSMITTED

Coding for this section required the use of mutually exclusive categories. Only manifest content in the text was used as evidence, and all three coders had to agree on the choice of category. There are eight categories in which the cause of HIV/AIDS transmission was coded: (1) heterosexual sex, (2) homosexual sex, (3) vertical transmission (mother to child), (4) intravenous drug use, (5) blood/blood products, (6) not known, (7) multiple risk factors, and (8) other. The data were examined with reference to gender and age.

Figure 2.2 summarizes the cause of infection by frequency. In many cases, the cause for HIV infection could not be identified. In fact, the largest single category, with 143 instances (38 percent), consists of characters whose cause of infection is not known. Of the identified causes of infection, heterosexual sex appears the most frequently: This is how 77 (20.5 percent) of the 376 characters contract HIV/AIDS. For 60 (16 percent) of the characters, homosexual sex is the next most frequently cited cause. Contaminated blood or blood products is responsible for

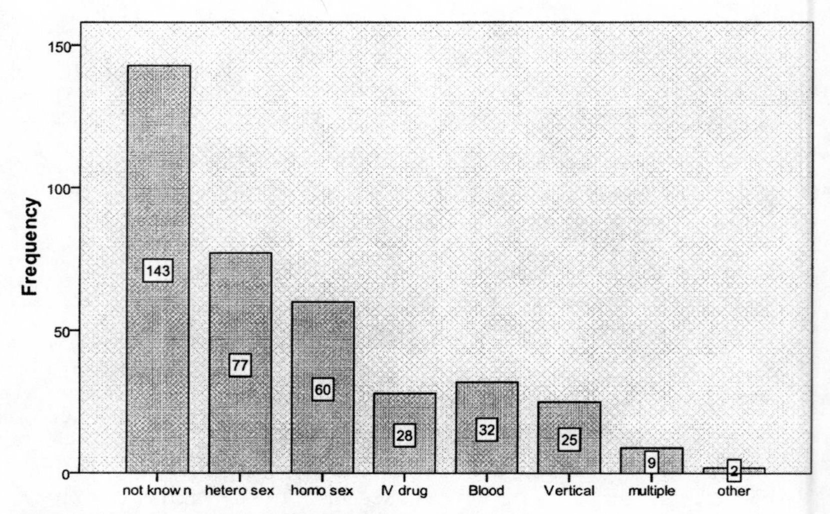

Figure 2.2. Cause of HIV/AIDS Transmission

32 (8.5 percent) of the infections. Intravenous drug use is next at 28 (7.4 percent), followed by vertical transmission at 25 (6.6 percent). Nine (2.4 percent) of the characters exhibit multiple risk factors and thus cannot be limited to a single cause. Two (0.5) fall into the catchall category of "other," which here refers to AIDS contracted as a result of a neural implant in a science fiction novel.

Gender

One way to consider HIV/AIDS infection is by gender. In general, males outnumber females in each category of infection. Within the most frequently coded category, "cause not known," there are 86 (60.1 percent) males, 30 (21 percent) females, and 27 (18.9 percent) persons of unknown gender. By gender overall, "cause not known" accounts for infection in 86 of 216 males (39.8 percent), 30 of 114 females (26.3 percent), and 27 of 46 individuals (58.7 percent) whose gender cannot be identified. The gender "unknown" vies with male and female in frequency in terms of the cause of infection in another category as well. Sixteen (50 percent) males, 4 (12.5 percent) females, and 12 (37.5 percent) persons of unknown gender contract HIV/AIDS by means of contaminated blood or blood products.

Homosexual sex is the cause of HIV/AIDS in 60 males, or 100 percent of the category. These 60 males comprise 27.8 percent of the males overall. There are no females who contract the disease through homosexual sex in the books.

In a small number of cases, infection may be attributed to multiple risks. Six (66.7 percent) of the males and 3 (33.3 percent) of the females are in this category.

There are some exceptions to the pattern of male dominance per category. Almost twice as many women as men contract HIV/AIDS through heterosexual sex: 26 (33.8 percent) males, 49 (63.6 percent) females, and 2 (2.6 percent) "unknown." Looking at gender overall, heterosexual sex is responsible for infection in 26 of 216 males (12 percent), 49 of 114 females (43 percent), and 2 of 46 characters (4.3 percent) whose gender is unknown. Similarly, more females than males acquire HIV/AIDS through vertical transmission: Twelve females (48 percent), 8 males (32 percent), and 5 (20 percent) persons of unknown gender contract the disease in this way. Slightly more females (15, or 53.6 percent) than males (13, or 46.4 percent) contract HIV/AIDS through intravenous drug use, but overall it is twice as frequent a cause of infection for 15 of 114 females (13.2 percent) than for 13 of 216 males (6 percent).

"Other" as a cause is distributed equally between males and females, with 1 (50 percent) male and 1 (50 percent) female contracting HIV/AIDS through a neural implant in a science fiction novel.

Age

This section provides a summary of the cause of infection by age category.

Nonviable Pregnancy and Young Child (Birth–Age 4)

The 2 cases (100 percent) in the category of nonviable pregnancy are miscarriages. The cause of infection is vertical transmission. Similarly, all 18 (94.7 percent) of the young children are infected through vertical transmission.

School-Age Child (Ages 5–10) and School-Age Child/Young Adult (Ages 5–19)

The most frequently cited cause of infection for the school-age children is "not known": For 6 (66.7 percent) of the characters, no reason is provided. Blood transfusions or blood products are responsible for 3 (33.3 percent) of the characters' illness. Again, for one (50 percent) character in the combined school-age child/young adult category, the cause of infection is not known; for the other one (50 percent), infected blood or blood products are deemed responsible.

Young Adult (Ages 11–19) and Young Adult/Emerging Adult (Ages 11–25)

Twenty-four (44.4 percent) of the young adult characters contract the disease through heterosexual sex. Seven (13 percent) of the characters contract the disease through blood or blood products; another 7 (13 percent) are infected by intravenous drug use. For 6 (11.1 percent) characters, the reason is not known. In 5 (9.3 percent) instances, homosexual sex is the next most frequently mentioned reason for infection. Three (5.6 percent) characters develop HIV/AIDS through vertical transmission. In 2 (3.7 percent) cases, the presence of multiple risks and lack of definitive manifest content do not allow a single reason for infection to emerge.

In the combined young adult/emerging adult category, no reason for the infection of 9 (64.3 percent) of the characters is provided. For 2 (14.3 percent) of the characters, the cause of infection is heterosexual sex. One (7.1 percent) character contracts HIV/AIDS through homosexual sex, a second (7.1 percent) from infected blood or blood products, and a third (7.1 percent) by means of multiple risk factors.

Emerging Adult (Ages 20–25) and Emerging Adult/Adult (Ages 20–64)

Three causes of infection appear most frequently among emerging adult characters: For 10 (30.3 percent) characters the cause is "unknown," while 9 (27.3 percent) characters contract the disease through homosexual sex, and in 8 (24.2 percent) cases the cause is heterosexual sex. Two (6.1 percent) of the characters are infected by intravenous drug use, and 2 (6.1 percent) characters are exposed to multiple risk factors. Blood or blood products and "other" causes account for 1 (3 percent) character each.

For 11 (39.3 percent) of the characters in this combined emerging adult/adult category, no reason is provided for the cause of infection. Nine (32.1 percent) of the characters contract the disease through homosexual sex, and 4 (14.3 percent) through heterosexual sex. In 3 (10.7 percent) of the cases, the reason provided is intravenous drug use. One (3.6 percent) of the characters is exposed to multiple risk factors.

Adult (Ages 26–64), Adult/Senior (Ages 26–65+), and Senior (Ages 65+)

In this adult category, the most frequent cause of infection is "not known." For 47 (32.2 percent) individuals no reason for infection is provided. Heterosexual sex is the cause of the disease for 37 (25.3 percent) of the characters and homosexual sex for 33 (22.6 percent) characters. Nineteen (13 percent) characters contract HIV/AIDS through blood or blood products. Six (4.1 percent) become ill through intravenous drug use. In 3 (2.1 percent) cases, multiple risks are involved. For 1 (0.7 percent) character, the reason is "other."

No cause of infection is attributed to the single (100 percent) character in the combined adult/senior category. No seniors with HIV/AIDS appear in the set of books.

Unknown

For 52 (75.4 percent) of the characters in this category, no indication of age or reason for infection is provided. In 10 (14.5 percent) cases, HIV-positive status is due to intravenous drug use. Three (4.3 percent) characters acquire HIV/AIDS through homosexual sex. Vertical transmission and heterosexual sex each account for 2 (2.9 percent) of the characters' illnesses.

DISCUSSION

This section discusses the implications of the findings and incorporates additional commentary to see how accurately a picture is drawn of who contracts HIV/AIDS and how the virus is transmitted in this set of novels.

Who Has HIV/AIDS?

In spite of improved treatments, youth ages thirteen to twenty-four years are at "persistent risk for HIV infection."[97] Even if young adults do not contract the disease themselves, people with HIV/AIDS are living longer, so young adults are more likely to know someone who does have it. The content analysis findings suggest that the books as a group do not do a good job of showing those connections, although individual books may do so.

A Close Relationship or No Relationship at All?

The largest group of characters with HIV/AIDS has no direct relationship to the protagonist. When just more than half of the characters are outside of the protagonists' circle of even casual acquaintances, the message being overwhelmingly sent by this set of books is that HIV/AIDS does not happen to people about whom the protagonist cares. It is a weakness of this literature that there are so few protagonists who themselves have HIV/AIDS. Young adult protagonists with HIV/AIDS appear sporadically in this body of literature, so there is unfortunately no indication that the occurrence of HIV-positive protagonists is increasing.

Although the majority of cases are people the protagonist does not know, some close connections such as family and friends are also likely to be struck by the disease in this set of novels. Most of the HIV-positive siblings are older and function as role models for the protagonist. Among extended family members, cousins and uncles are the ones with the closest emotional ties to the protagonist. The few aunts are just mentioned in passing, and grandparents are noticeably absent.

Seniors are in short supply. That there is only a single adult/senior depicted as having HIV/AIDS in the books is due to the way the coding was applied to the data. For example, two seniors were noted but not coded because the researchers would have had to bring in information that was supplemental to the text. Thus the ages of celebrities Rock Hudson and Liberace in *Until Whatever* could have been determined, but only by using information a reader would not find in the narrative.[98] Although seniors are barely in evidence in this set of books, the Centers for Disease Control and Prevention report that the number of persons ages fifty and over with HIV/AIDS is increasing. This is due in part to improved treatments and in part to newly diagnosed cases.[99] Greater visibility of HIV-positive seniors in this literature would be more true to life.

Friends with HIV/AIDS do appear in this set of books. More of these friends are male than female, with both genders fairly evenly distributed through the years of publication. Three of the friends are adults, all gay males: Cosmo Farber in *Touch of the Clown*,[100] Josiah Stemp in *Zach at Risk*,[101] and Daphne/Eddie in *When Love Comes to Town*.[102] Assuming that young adult readers will gravitate most strongly to characters in their own age group and other people close to them, then this subset of the overall group of novels communicates that HIV/AIDS is indeed a disease that could strike them or their friends or family.

Family friends can also be close. Interestingly, only in the novels with an African setting does a "family friend" with HIV/AIDS appear: Mrs. Tafa's son, Emmanuel, in *Chanda's Secrets*;[103] Binti's grandmother's friend, Jeremiah, in *The Heaven Shop*;[104] most of the Malapa family in *Far and Beyon'*;[105] and the Malungas in *Chanda's Wars*.[106]

Paying Attention to HIV/AIDS

Though an urgent public health issue in the West, the reality of HIV/AIDS is best communicated in the books set in Africa and Papua New Guinea. It is in these books in particular that the "uncountable" indications of people in hospitals and graveyards is most apparent. The use of statistics to emphasize the magnitude of the problem is also commonplace. Staggering statistics appear in *The Heaven Shop*: "Eighty percent of the people who come into this hospital have AIDS. . . . Thirty percent of the people in our cities are HIV positive, almost half of Malawi's civil servants are HIV positive, and our health care workers and our teachers are dying of AIDS faster than they can be replaced."[107] In *Playing with Fire*, a local doctor outlines the situation of young people across Mozambique: "'Just now, during the few minutes we're sitting here talking together, other young people are catching the infection,' Dr. Nkeka said."[108] Or, as succinctly stated in *Far and Beyon'*, "Too much death was deadening emotions."[109] In *The Silent Killer*, Natasha's Barbadian youth group faces a daunting challenge; in an effort to "facilitate sufferers and their families, helping people to cope with the disease, dying and death. . . . We hoped in the future to raise enough money to build another hostel for sufferers."[110] The situation is also overwhelming in *Notes from a Spinning Planet: Papua New Guinea*: Maddie's aunt says, "When it comes to the subject of the AIDS epidemic in Papua New Guinea, people seem to just throw up their hands and shake their heads like it's hopeless."[111] Such books communicate the dramatic impact of HIV/AIDS on these countries, but this focus can overshadow the realization that HIV/AIDS is of epidemic proportions in the United States as well.

However, some books set in such developed countries as the United States also use statistics to build a sense of urgency about HIV/AIDS. In *The Mayday Rampage*, rapidly increasing AIDS statistics for 1988 through 1992 build to the following statement: "After more than 12 years, more than 250,000 diagnosed cases, and more than 160,000 deaths of AIDS in the United States, there is finally hope for a national plan of action against AIDS."[112] Looking up prevalence rates is important for Robin in *Robin's Diary* as she grapples with her partner Stone's HIV-positive diagnosis: "According to my notes, there have been 441,528 cases of AIDS diagnosed and reported since 1981. Of those, 270,870 individuals have died—leaving 170,658 currently living with AIDS."[113] Chris, in *Beyond the Wind*, shares with his friend Jen the frightening statistics that he has discovered: "Did you know that 33 million people are living with HIV? And did you know that based on what scientists know, five young people are infected every minute, which results in 7,000 new cases per day, and half of those people are fifteen to twenty-four years of age?"[114] In *Rumors and Whispers*, a school board member informs the audience at a public meeting of the reported number of infections among young people: "The Centers for Disease Control in Atlanta says there are 415 cases of AIDS among kids from ages 13 to 19. That's a 40-percent increase in the last 2 years. And that's for *reported* cases."[115]

The issue of AIDS orphans is a recurring theme in the books set in Africa. For example, in *Playing with Fire*: "'So many are dying,' Graçieta cried. 'This disease will empty our villages. Soon there'll only be children and old folk left. What will happen then?'"[116] In *The Heaven Shop*, Binti is amazed to see all the children when she arrives at her grandmother's cattle post: "There were at least 200 children in the yard."[117] Binti's grandmother, Gogo, explains how all the AIDS orphans she cares for are, in one way or another, cousins and therefore part of their extended family. Even if the orphans survive, it is in the midst of seeing their families decimated by HIV/AIDS, as noted in *Far and Beyon'*: "So many dying. So many children watching as their loved ones waste away and die."[118]

However, it is not just in the African narratives that AIDS orphans appear. A number of the books set in the developed world also feature young people who have lost one or both parents to AIDS. In *Woman Soldier/La Soldadera*, Nico's parents both die of AIDS, and from the age of five onward she is raised by her grandparents.[119] Similarly, in *One True Friend*, Amir's parents both succumb to AIDS, but he ends up in foster care.[120] Will's father dies of AIDS at the end of *Strays Like Us*,[121] and an initially reluctant Janie in *Born Blue* cares for her mother until Mama Linda passes away.[122] In *Something Terrible Happened*, Gillian's mother deteriorates rapidly and dies.[123]

"Uncountable" indications of people with HIV/AIDS form the backdrop for fifty-two books. The presence of such AIDS services as hotlines, dedicated clinics, support groups, and activity around the AIDS quilt demonstrate that the epidemic is ongoing in developed countries, too. *Zach at Risk* describes the situation for HIV-positive gay men in Seattle: "AIDS services were just getting started in Seattle that year as hundreds of men like Josiah began to get ill and start their slow, terrible dying."[124] In *I Never Got to Say Good-Bye*, while trying to muster volunteers to help build support for an AIDS hospice the community does not want, Traci refers to a hotline: "Did you read about the Teen-AIDS Hotline? Maybe we could start one."[125] In *Rumors and Whispers*, Sarah wonders about the AIDS clinic she and David are visiting: "As they walked past each empty room, she noticed a sign outside the doors announcing that AIDS patients occupied those rooms, and she winced thinking how hard it must be to be reminded of this every time you came in or out of your room."[126] Emma is relieved to discover that her support group in *The Beat Goes On* "was a room full of people just like me who either had HIV or knew someone in their family who had it."[127] In *Tommy Stands Alone*, Tommy and his counselor Sonia "walked around speechless amidst the throngs of people who had come from all over the central coast of California to pay tribute to the people whose faces and names were on the panels of the quilt."[128]

In some books the reader might expect to see "uncountables" in the background but none exist. For example, the milieu of *The Tragedy of Miss Geneva Flowers* is rife with such high-risk behaviors as intravenous drug use and unprotected sex, yet surprisingly there is no mention of AIDS hotlines or support groups.[129]

How Did They Get It?

The following section discusses the different reasons for HIV/AIDS infection and how they are portrayed in this set of books, beginning with "cause not known," the most frequently coded cause.

Cause Not Known

No information is provided to explain how the largest single group of characters acquire HIV/AIDS. Included here are mostly marginal characters who the protagonist knows only slightly, if at all. Examples of such characters are the patients in the AIDS ward in *Rumors and Whispers*[130] and various patients at the hospital in *The Heaven Shop*.[131] It is usually impossible to identify how a blood donor who passes the disease on to a character through infected blood contracted it himself or herself, so "not known" is the only reasonable code to apply. As noted above, if the actual cause of infection for celebrities was not mentioned in the text and thus not manifestly communicated to the reader, it was coded as "not known."

Surprisingly, how the disease is acquired is not explained for some HIV-positive characters the protagonist knows very well. One example is Crystal's Uncle Joe in *Life Magic*, where Crystal is not told (and does not ask) how he got HIV/AIDS.[132] In *What about Anna?*, the reader is not told how Anna's now dead brother Jonas contracted the disease.[133] Not identifying the cause may add a touch of mystery to the novel, but it leaves out information that is crucial to understanding the transmission of HIV/AIDS.

Heterosexual Sex

Though "cause not known" is the most frequently encountered code for HIV/AIDS transmission in this set of books, the most common identified cause of infection is heterosexual sex. For females, it is the most likely way to acquire the disease. In the novels set in Africa, it is not unusual for parents or stepparents to have HIV/AIDS, as shown in *Chanda's Secrets*,[134] *The Heaven Shop*,[135] and *The Girl Who Saw Lions*.[136] Heterosexual sex is the most common means of transmission in the Sub-Saharan countries where these books are set. For the books that take place in the United States, circumstances may differ, but the cause is the same. Claire's parents in *The Deeper, the Bluer* both contract HIV/AIDS, Vince by having an affair with a male actor and then passing it on to his wife, Virginia.[137] In the case of Nico's parents, Alex and Miranda, in *Woman Soldier/La Soldadera*, Alex gives it to Miranda during a conjugal visit.[138]

The situation of poor women in Sub-Saharan African countries has particular ramifications related to HIV/AIDS. Inequalities within the family, violence against women, and women's inheritance and property rights all conspire to make women more vulnerable to infection.[139] Many women turn to survival sex, engaging in sex for payment or economic support within an abusive relationship so they can care for their families in situations where there are few other options. Since men paying for sex often do not want to use protection and in prostitution multiple partners are involved, the risk of HIV/AIDS infection is very high. This is Junie's situation in *The Heaven Shop*: "Men pay more if she doesn't make them use a condom."[140] In *Chanda's Secrets*, Esther supports her siblings by working as a prostitute after the death of her parents from AIDS, but she cannot continue when she is attacked, raped, and contracts HIV/AIDS herself.[141] Sometimes protection is not used because the character does not know any better. Uneducated Rosa in *Playing with Fire* "had made love with four different boys. . . . Dr. Nkeka said that in Rosa's case, Steven was the most likely source of infection. . . . Had the boys used any protection when they made love? Rosa had just shaken her head. She had only the vaguest idea of what he was taking about."[142]

Living in a developed country, however, is no guarantee that characters use protection when having sex. Precious, the illiterate HIV-positive young adult victim of incest in *Push*, with one child by her father and another on the way, has few resources to draw upon in an inner-city nightmare of sexual violence.[143] In *What You Don't Know Can Kill You*, Ellen is educated but still naïve enough to believe that she is in a monogamous relationship with her boyfriend, Jack.[144] It turns out that Jack does not think a fraternity night spent with prostitutes amounts to infidelity: "And they brought in girls, you know, girls from town. No one even knew them—it wasn't like making love, Ellie. It was—it was—you know, just sex. . . . I didn't even have any condoms."[145]

Homosexual Sex

Books in which homosexual sex is identified as a cause of HIV/AIDS are fairly evenly distributed from 1986 through 2008. This method of transmission is limited to males; no females contract HIV/AIDS through homosexual sex even though there are lesbians in the books, for example, Zach's mom and her partner in *Zach at Risk*.[146] No HIV-positive protagonists are gay, although, as noted above, there are gay friends with HIV/AIDS. The homosexual characters with HIV/AIDS most closely related to the protagonist are fathers, brothers, and uncles as well as such role models as teachers or older friends. Many are in committed monogamous relationships with a partner who is dying or dead. In *The Mayday Rampage*, Jess and Molly's teacher, Mr. Goodban, lives with his partner Vic, who is ill.[147] When Barbara and Livvy visit their gay adult friend, Cosmo, in *Touch of the Clown*, they see a photo of his partner, Roberto, who died of AIDS.[148] Similarly, Jack's lover, Lincoln, in *My Brother Has AIDS*, is already dead when the novel begins.[149] Unusually, Philip's lover, Geoff, in *The Eagle Kite* is relegated to the background because Philip is still in the closet.[150] Philip's son, Liam, the protagonist, therefore has to cope both with Philip's failing health and the revelation that his father is gay.

Intravenous Drug Use

Considering the strong likelihood of needle-sharing among intravenous drug users and the popularity of steroid use among athletes, it is surprising that so few instances of this method of transmission are depicted in the books. Monk, the student athlete in *Get It While It's Hot. Or Not*, and the "muscle-head" with whom he shares a needle provide the only examples of steroid use resulting in HIV/AIDS.[151] There are more instances of characters participating in unspecified intravenous drug use and needle-sharing, including in *A Dream to Cherish*,[152] when Arien and another person share a needle, as well as use by the guitar player and drummer in *What Happened to Lani Garver*.[153]

Of particular note is the phenomenon of mothers who contract HIV/AIDS in this way, although this is largely in part due to a single book, *Baby Alicia Is Dying*, in which there are seven drug-addict mothers whose babies are born with HIV.[154] Another such baby, Melody, appears in *The Case of the Missing Melody*,[155] and its sequel, *The Mystery of the Poison Pen*.[156] But Holden's mother in *Dream Water*[157] is also an addict, as are both of Amir's late parents in *One True Friend*.[158]

Blood/Blood Products

Formerly a legitimate cause of HIV/AIDS, it is now extremely unlikely that anyone would contract the disease through an infected blood transfusion or blood product, since the blood supply has been safe since 1985. Nevertheless, books that provide this as the explanation were published as late as 2004. Josh, a hemophiliac in *Diving for the Moon*,[159] contracts HIV/AIDS through a tainted blood product, as does David Deering in *The Mayday Rampage*.[160] Typically, however, the person with HIV/AIDS has been given a blood transfusion with infected blood during surgery after a near-fatal car accident. This is the case for Anne in *Sixteen and Dying*[161] and Kimberly in *Losing David*.[162]

In two cases, a tainted blood transfusion is used by parents as a more socially acceptable reason to hide the real cause of transmission. In *Fade to Black*, Alex's mother tells everyone her teenaged son has contracted HIV/AIDS from a blood transfusion rather than admit the cause is heterosexual sex.[163] In *The Eagle Kite*, Liam's parents conspire to tell him that his father (who is not openly gay) acquired HIV/AIDS through a transfusion rather than through homosexual sex.[164]

Another notable way in which the disease is transmitted is through needlesticks in a medical setting. *Rumors and Whispers* refers to twelve medical workers who contract HIV/AIDS in this manner.[165] Although precautions can be taken to minimize the risk of transmission, it is still a possibility.

Vertical Transmission

In this set of books, vertical (mother to child) transmission is a cause of HIV/AIDS for both children and young adults. Most of the children in this selection of books are babies born with HIV. They appear in *Baby Alicia Is Dying,*[166] *The Case of the Missing Melody,*[167] *The Mystery of the Poison Pen,*[168] and most of the novels set in Africa. There are also some school-age children, for example, Pilada's two children in *Notes from a Spinning Planet: Papua New Guinea.*[169] Since people are now living longer with HIV/AIDS, it is not surprising to find young adults in this category. Three young adults appear in two of the more recent books: Ellie in *The Beat Goes On*[170] and Cleo and Gabe in *Soul Love.*[171]

The circumstances in which children with vertical transmission live vary greatly. In general, children in the African books do not have much of a chance to survive, let alone thrive, whereas in the developed countries, young adults with good medical care and support can live with HIV/AIDS much as one would manage a chronic illness. This stark contrast underlines the economic realities of HIV/AIDS: Treatment must be affordable and available for children infected through vertical transmission to have any real future.

Multiple Risk Factors

Young adults are not unacquainted with risky behaviors, but they may not associate them directly with HIV/AIDS. In *Night Kites,* for example, Erick does not seem to realize that unprotected sex with Nikki, who used to sleep with an intravenous drug user, is very risky indeed.[172] A combination of needle-sharing and unprotected sex, as in the case of the unnamed haggard young adult in *Of Cause and Consequence,* is typical of the multiple risk factors in this set of books.[173] Greater awareness of the implications of these behaviors in this body of literature would provide the reader with much-needed information.

Other

In one book, the science fiction novel *Singing the Dogstar Blues,* there are two characters who acquire HIV/AIDS by means of a neural implant.[174] The surgery enhances brain power at the risk of contracting HIV/AIDS. How poignant and sad that, as the AIDS museum director says, "People don't learn, do they?"[175] The mere fact that a science fiction novelist would choose to write about HIV/AIDS not just as a disease of the past but as one that continues into the future suggests the power and pull of HIV/AIDS as a literary subject.

SUMMARY AND CONCLUSIONS

This chapter considers two research questions: who has HIV/AIDS and how did they acquire it? Findings regarding the HIV-positive characters' relationship to the protagonist, their gender, and their age are presented. The causes of infection are enumerated and considered in terms of gender and age. A general discussion sets the findings within the context of what is known about HIV/AIDS and how accurately these books depict that information. Although the books as a whole may not reflect the immediacy of HIV/AIDS in the lives of young adults, some books do communicate the true nature of the epidemic and provide accurate information about who can become HIV positive and how that occurs.

Since more than half of the HIV-positive characters are individuals with whom the young adult protagonist has no direct relationship, it cannot be said that young adults are likely to feel great empathy for them. However, the presence of immediate and extended family members, friends, and even HIV-positive protagonists themselves do offer many examples of characters close to the young adult protagonist and so are likely to generate greater interest and empathy. In terms of gender, HIV/AIDS is no longer depicted as an exclusively adult male problem, but it is now one in which more often young adults themselves are directly involved. Although there is no trend toward an increasing number of young adult protagonists who are HIV positive, a larger number of younger HIV-positive characters, often friends of the protagonist, do appear in the books.

An accurate picture of the pandemic in many books is bolstered by the use of "uncountables," indications that, along with the use of statistics, describe the backdrop against which the narrative plays out in the books set in Sub-Saharan Africa and Papua New Guinea. Although the seriousness of the situation in these countries tends to overshadow all else, some (although not many) of the books set in the developed world successfully use these devices to communicate the urgency of the epidemic here as well. Occasionally books set in the developed countries do not contain "uncountables" where one would expect to find them, that is, in a high-risk milieu.

The largest single cause of HIV/AIDS infection in these books is "cause not known." In some cases not even the cause of infection of someone close to the protagonist is revealed. This is a lost opportunity to provide important information to young adult readers.

Heterosexual sex is the largest identified cause of infection and has a particular impact on females, especially in Sub-Saharan Africa. The patterns of infection in these books accurately reflect the phenomenon of survival sex and the special burden that HIV/AIDS places on females. Infection through homosexual sex in this set of books is limited to males. The inclusion of lesbians would make the picture of who contracts HIV through homosexual sex more balanced.

The incidence of intravenous drug use in the novels, especially steroid use, is not as high as might be expected considering that this is a serious risk factor for HIV/AIDS. This picture does not reflect reality and would serve young readers better if needle-sharing were shown more often as the cause of infection. On the other hand, tainted blood and blood products have not been genuine risk factors for HIV/AIDS infection since 1985, when the blood supply was declared safe, yet a good number of these books, all published after 1985, still portray blood transfusions and products as a viable cause of HIV/AIDS. A tainted blood transfusion is even sometimes used as a more socially acceptable excuse to hide the true source of infection.

Vertical transmission no longer refers simply to babies and young children who are unlikely to survive, although such characters are certainly in evidence. Children born with HIV who receive proper medical care are living longer, healthier lives. This is reflected in the set of books, as both school-age children and young adults with HIV/AIDS make an appearance. There is a marked difference in treatment options and health outcomes for these youth in developing and developed countries.

A fairly small number of infections are attributable to such multiple risk factors as multiple sex partners and needle-sharing.

More emphasis on these behaviors would paint a clearer picture of the true risks. As for "other" causes, the science fiction novel *Singing the Dogstar Blues* posits a risky neural implant that brings with it the possibility of AIDS.[176]

Ideally the protagonist should see HIV/AIDS as a genuine threat that affects people for whom he or she cares, transmitted in a way that is not only possible but probable. When the protagonist has strong emotional ties to the HIV-positive character and must cope with the disease close to home, the stage is set for greater engagement and empathy. The gender and age of the character with HIV/AIDS can also influence the protagonist's reactions. Such verisimilitude provides for accurate and accessible HIV/AIDS information in a young adult–friendly source. However, when more than half of the HIV-positive characters have no direct relationship to the protagonist and the most frequently cited cause of infection is "cause not known," the sense of connection is lessened and not as much of this vital information is available to readers.

NOTES

1. Angela Elwell Hunt, *A Dream to Cherish*, Cassie Perkins Series, No. 4 (Lincoln, NE: Authors Guild Backinprint.com Edition/iUniverse .com, 1992), 122.
2. Centers for Disease Control and Prevention (CDC), "HIV and Its Transmission," 1999 (last reviewed by the CDC on March 8, 2007). Available at www.cdc.gov/hiv/resources/factsheets/transmission.htm (18 November 2009).
3. Deborah Ellis, *The Heaven Shop* (Allston, MA: Fitzhenry & Whiteside, 2004).
4. Clayton Bess, *The Mayday Rampage* (Sacramento, CA: Lookout Press, 1993).
5. Bess, *The Mayday Rampage.*
6. Alice Hoffman, *At Risk* (New York: Putnam, 1988).
7. Alex Flinn, *Fade to Black* (New York: HarperTempest, 2005).
8. Allan Stratton, *Chanda's Secrets* (New York: Annick Press, 2004).
9. Gayle Roper, *The Case of the Missing Melody*, East Edge Mysteries, No. 4 (Elgin, IL: Chariot Books/David C. Cook Publishing Co., 1993).
10. Ellis, *The Heaven Shop.*
11. Karen Rivers, *Dream Water* (Custer, WA: Orca Book Publishers, 1999).
12. Alison Goodman, *Singing the Dogstar Blues* (New York: Viking, 2002).

13. M. E. Kerr, *Night Kites* (New York: HarperTrophy, 1986).
14. Deborah Davis, *My Brother Has AIDS* (New York: Jean Karl/Atheneum, 1994).
15. Unity Dow, *Far and Beyon'* (San Francisco: Aunt Lute Books, 2001).
16. Henning Mankell, *Playing with Fire*, trans. from Swedish by Anna Paterson (Crows Nest, NSW, Australia: Allen & Unwin, 2002).
17. Fran Arrick, *What You Don't Know Can Kill You* (New York: Bantam Books, 1992).
18. Stratton, *Chanda's Secrets.*
19. Alida E. Young, *I Never Got to Say Good-Bye* (Worthington, OH: Willowisp Press, 1988).
20. Gregory Maguire, *Oasis* (New York: Clarion Books, 1996).
21. Adele Minchin, *The Beat Goes On* (New York: Simon & Schuster, 2004).
22. Bess, *The Mayday Rampage.*
23. Marilyn Levy, *Rumors and Whispers* (New York: Fawcett Juniper/Ballantine Books, 1990).
24. Jane Breskin Zalben, *Unfinished Dreams* (New York: Simon & Schuster Books for Young Readers, 1996).
25. Barbara Chase, *The Silent Killer* (Kingston, Jamaica: Ian Randle Publishers, 2005).
26. Tom Lennon, *When Love Comes to Town* (Dublin: O'Brien Press, 1993).
27. Glen Huser, *Touch of the Clown* (Buffalo, NY: Groundwood, 1999).
28. Stephanie Perry Moore, *Laurel Shadrach Series 2: Totally Free* (Chicago: Moody Press, 2002).
29. Stephanie Perry Moore, *Laurel Shadrach Series 3: Equally Yoked* (Chicago: Moody Publishers, 2003).
30. Stephanie Perry Moore, *Laurel Shadrach Series 4: Absolutely Worthy* (Chicago: Moody Publishers, 2003).
31. Stephanie Perry Moore, *Laurel Shadrach Series 5: Finally Sure* (Chicago: Moody Publishers, 2004).
32. Flinn, *Fade to Black.*
33. Charlotte St. John, *Red Hair Three* (New York: Fawcett Juniper, 1992).
34. Judith Pinsker, *Robin's Diary* (Radnor, PA: ABC Daytime Press/Chilton Book Company, 1995).
35. Alex Sanchez, *Rainbow Boys* (New York: Simon & Schuster, 2001).
36. Alex Sanchez, *Rainbow High* (New York: Simon Pulse, 2003).
37. Alex Sanchez, *Rainbow Road* (New York: Simon & Schuster, 2005).

38. Stratton, *Chanda's Secrets.*

39. Dow, *Far and Beyon'.*

40. Patricia Hermes, *Be Still My Heart* (New York: G. P. Putnam's Sons, 1989).

41. Bess, *The Mayday Rampage.*

42. Davis, *My Brother Has AIDS.*

43. Flinn, *Fade to Black.*

44. Lurlene McDaniel, *Baby Alicia Is Dying* (New York: Bantam, 1993).

45. Stratton, *Chanda's Secrets.*

46. Minchin, *The Beat Goes On.*

47. Lutz Van Dijk, *Stronger than the Storm,* trans. Karin Chubb (Cape Town: Maskew Miller Longman Pty., Ltd., 2000).

48. Todd Strasser, *Can't Get There from Here* (New York: Simon & Schuster, 2004).

49. Roper, *The Case of the Missing Melody.*

50. Gayle Roper, *The Mystery of the Poison Pen,* East Edge Mysteries, No. 5 (Elgin, IL: Chariot Books/David C. Cook Publishing Co., 1994).

51. Lee F. Bantle, *Diving for the Moon* (New York: Macmillan Books for Young Readers, 1995), 110.

52. Martha Humphreys, *Until Whatever* (New York: Clarion Books, 1991).

53. Stephanie Perry Moore, *Laurel Shadrach Series 1: Purity Reigns* (Chicago: Moody Press, 2002), 208.

54. Paula Fox, *The Eagle Kite* (New York: Orchard Books, 1995).

55. Arrick, *What You Don't Know Can Kill You.*

56. Davis, *My Brother Has AIDS.*

57. Strasser, *Can't Get There from Here.*

58. Maguire, *Oasis.*

59. Ellis, *The Heaven Shop.*

60. Flinn, *Fade to Black.*

61. Lurlene McDaniel, *Sixteen and Dying* (One Last Wish) (New York: Bantam, 1992).

62. Cherie Bennett and Jeff Gottesfeld, *University Hospital: Heart Trauma,* Book Four (New York: Berkley Jam Books, 2000).

63. Francesca Lia Block, *I Was a Teenage Fairy* (New York: Joanna Cotler Books/HarperCollins, 1998).

64. Jack Womack, *Random Acts of Senseless Violence* (New York: Atlantic Monthly Press, 1994).

65. Bess, *The Mayday Rampage.*

66. Humphreys, *Until Whatever.*

67. Jan Simoen, *What about Anna?,* trans. from Dutch by John Nieuwenhuizen (New York: Walker & Company, 2002).

68. Rex Harley, *Now That I've Found You* (Llandysul, Ceredigion, Wales: Pont Books/Gomer Press, 2003).

69. Hunt, *A Dream to Cherish*.
70. Ellis, *The Heaven Shop*.
71. Levy, *Rumors and Whispers*.
72. Young, *I Never Got to Say Good-Bye*.
73. Gloria Velásquez, *Tommy Stands Alone* (Houston, TX: Piñata Books/Arte Público Press, 1995), 123.
74. Pamela Shepherd, *Zach at Risk* (New York: Alice Street Editions/ Haworth Press, 2004), 174.
75. Pinsker, *Robin's Diary*, 122.
76. Melody Carlson, *Notes from a Spinning Planet: Papua New Guinea* (Colorado Springs, CO: WaterBrook Press/Random House, 2007), 199–200.
77. AVERT, "Women, HIV, and AIDS," 2009. Available at www.avert .org/women-hiv-aids.htm (9 October 2009).
78. Carlson, *Notes from a Spinning Planet: Papua New Guinea*, 73.
79. Lynda Waterhouse, *Soul Love* (London: Piccadilly Press, 2004).
80. Valerie Hobbs, *Get It While It's Hot. Or Not* (New York: Richard Jackson/Orchard, 1996), 146.
81. Hoffman, *At Risk*.
82. McDaniel, *Sixteen and Dying*.
83. Young, *I Never Got to Say Good-Bye*.
84. Bantle, *Diving for the Moon*.
85. Levy, *Rumors and Whispers*.
86. Eve Eliot, *Insatiable: The Compelling Story of Four Teens, Food, and Its Power* (Deerfield Beach, FL: Health Communications, 2001), 35.
87. Bess, *The Mayday Rampage*.
88. Melrose Cooper, *Life Magic* (New York: Henry Holt and Company, 1996).
89. Block, *I Was a Teenage Fairy*, 144.
90. Fox, *The Eagle Kite*, 2.
91. Fox, *The Eagle Kite*, 4.
92. Han Nolan, *Born Blue* (New York: Harcourt, 2001).
93. Diana Wieler, *Ran Van: Magic Nation* (Buffalo, NY: Groundwood Books/Douglas & McIntyre, 1997).
94. Wieler, *Ran Van*, 188.
95. Sapphire, *Push* (New York: Vintage Contemporaries, 1996), 150.
96. Goodman, *Singing the Dogstar Blues*, 23–24.
97. Centers for Disease Control and Prevention (CDC), "HIV/AIDS among Youth," revised August 2008. Available at www.cdc.gov/hiv/ pubs/facts/youth.htm (18 November 2009).
98. Humphreys, *Until Whatever*.
99. Centers for Disease Control and Prevention (CDC), "HIV/AIDS among Persons Aged 50 and Older," revised February 2008. Available at www.cdc.gov/hiv/topics/over50/resources/factsheets/over50.htm (15 October 2009).

100. Huser, *Touch of the Clown.*
101. Shepherd, *Zach at Risk.*
102. Lennon, *When Love Comes to Town.*
103. Stratton, *Chanda's Secrets.*
104. Ellis, *The Heaven Shop.*
105. Dow, *Far and Beyon'.*
106. Allan Stratton, *Chanda's Wars* (New York: HarperTeen, 2008).
107. Ellis, *The Heaven Shop*, 53.
108. Mankell, *Playing with Fire*, 180.
109. Dow, *Far and Beyon'*, 26.
110. Chase, *The Silent Killer*, 101.
111. Carlson, *Notes from a Spinning Planet: Papua New Guinea*, 22.
112. Bess, *The Mayday Rampage*, 198.
113. Pinsker, *Robin's Diary*, 122.
114. Rob N. Hood, *Beyond the Wind* (Binghamton, NY: Southern Tier Editions/Harrington Park Press/Haworth Press, 2004), 217.
115. Levy, *Rumors and Whispers*, 146.
116. Mankell, *Playing with Fire*, 199.
117. Ellis, *The Heaven Shop*, 128.
118. Dow, *Far and Beyon'*, 168.
119. Irene Beltrán Hernández, *Woman Soldier/La Soldadera* (Waco, TX: Blue Rose Books, 1998).
120. Joyce Hansen, *One True Friend* (New York: Clarion, 2001).
121. Richard Peck, *Strays Like Us* (New York: Puffin Books, 1998).
122. Nolan, *Born Blue.*
123. Barbara Ann Porte, *Something Terrible Happened* (New York: Orchard Books, 1994).
124. Shepherd, *Zach at Risk*, 130.
125. Young, *I Never Got to Say Good-Bye*, 161.
126. Levy, *Rumors and Whispers*, 125.
127. Minchin, *The Beat Goes On*, 71.
128. Velásquez, *Tommy Stands Alone*, 123.
129. Joe Babcock, *The Tragedy of Miss Geneva Flowers* (New York: Carroll & Graf Publishers, 2005).
130. Levy, *Rumors and Whispers.*
131. Ellis, *The Heaven Shop.*
132. Cooper, *Life Magic.*
133. Simoen, *What about Anna?*
134. Stratton, *Chanda's Secrets.*
135. Ellis, *The Heaven Shop.*
136. Berlie Doherty, *The Girl Who Saw Lions* (New York: Neal Porter/Roaring Brook Press, 2008).
137. Barbara Field, *The Deeper, the Bluer* (Lincoln, NE: iUniverse.com, 2000).
138. Hernández, *Woman Soldier/La Soldadera.*

139. AVERT, "Women, HIV, and AIDS."
140. Ellis, *The Heaven Shop*, 170.
141. Stratton, *Chanda's Secrets*.
142. Mankell, *Playing with Fire*, 125.
143. Sapphire, *Push*.
144. Arrick, *What You Don't Know Can Kill You*.
145. Arrick, *What You Don't Know Can Kill You*, 56.
146. Shepherd, *Zach at Risk*.
147. Bess, *The Mayday Rampage*.
148. Huser, *Touch of the Clown*.
149. Davis, *My Brother Has AIDS*.
150. Fox, *The Eagle Kite*.
151. Hobbs, *Get It While It's Hot. Or Not*.
152. Hunt, *A Dream to Cherish*.
153. Carol Plum-Ucci, *What Happened to Lani Garver* (Orlando, FL: Harcourt, 2002).
154. McDaniel, *Baby Alicia Is Dying*.
155. Roper, *The Case of the Missing Melody*.
156. Roper, *The Mystery of the Poison Pen*.
157. Rivers, *Dream Water*.
158. Hansen, *One True Friend*.
159. Bantle, *Diving for the Moon*.
160. Bess, *The Mayday Rampage*.
161. McDaniel, *Sixteen and Dying*.
162. Elizabeth Benning, *Losing David* (New York: Harper Paperbacks, 1994).
163. Flinn, *Fade to Black*.
164. Fox, *The Eagle Kite*.
165. Levy, *Rumors and Whispers*.
166. McDaniel, *Baby Alicia Is Dying*.
167. Roper, *The Case of the Missing Melody*.
168. Roper, *The Mystery of the Poison Pen*.
169. Carlson, *Notes from a Spinning Planet: Papua New Guinea*.
170. Minchin, *The Beat Goes On*.
171. Waterhouse, *Soul Love*.
172. Kerr, *Night Kites*.
173. Alida Scheiderer, *Of Cause and Consequence* (Scotts Valley, CA: CreateSpace, 2008).
174. Goodman, *Singing the Dogstar Blues*.
175. Goodman, *Singing the Dogstar Blues*, 130.
176. Goodman, *Singing the Dogstar Blues*.

3

What Are We Afraid of? Protagonist Views of Risk

> "*Excuse me,* but I don't want *that* guy's skin particles on me."
>
> —Alex Flinn, *Fade to Black*[1]

The fears about HIV that a protagonist expresses provide, ideally, a means of conveying the risk factors related to HIV/AIDS to an audience of young adult readers. To that end, this chapter seeks to answer the question, What are the explicit fears of protagonists regarding HIV/AIDS?, and the extent to which this body of literature addresses fears surrounding HIV/AIDS is examined in this section. Because HIV is not only a biomedical but also a sociocultural problem, fears regarding such issues as social isolation, violence, and loss of control are discussed alongside those related to physical risk factors for contracting the disease.

Protagonist fears are addressed in terms of whether fear messages are present in the narrative at all, or whether there is manifest content that the protagonist has no fear. Also discussed are those instances where a protagonist is unsure whether he or she is afraid. Finally, explicit manifest fears are examined in terms of whether the protagonist fears for himself or herself or for others.

When a protagonist explicitly experiences fear, these fears are further examined as to whether they are reasonable or unreasonable. For example, a protagonist might have a reasonable fear of contracting HIV after having unprotected sex, as Nelson does in *Rainbow Boys*.[2] Likewise, he or she might unreasonably fear for a family member who visits the house of someone who has HIV, like Clinton in *Fade to Black*.[3] Unreasonable fears are defined as any fears expressed about contracting the disease in the absence of true risk factors, and they are most commonly expressed as fears of varying levels of casual contact. Reasonable fears are defined as those that reflect true risk factors for the disease, including unprotected sex and intravenous drug use.

Management of risk is an important factor to consider when determining whether a fear is reasonable or unreasonable. For instance, HIV can be contracted via contaminated blood. This kind of exposure is, therefore, a reasonable fear. However, in *At Risk*, the parents at school worry that Amanda, who is infected with HIV, will bleed on the uneven bars in gym practice and that one of the other children will get that blood into a blister and contract HIV.[4] While this could indeed happen in the absence of any precautions, there are many very simple precautions that could be taken to avoid transmission of HIV in these circumstances.

While coding, a distinction was made between fear specifically of AIDS or HIV versus fear of death, loss, or suffering. For example, in *My Brother Has AIDS*, Lacy feels fear when she sees her brother for the first time after his diagnosis, but the fear is related to Jack having "withdrawn into his own body," and she discusses wanting to reach him and draw him back out.[5] It was deemed that this was fear of loss and not specifically of AIDS. At another point in the same novel, however, Lacy states that, "Even though I know I won't catch it, I sometimes picture tiny viruses flying around the room, somehow escaping and leaping onto me or into a little cut on my finger that I hadn't noticed."[6] In this instance, Lacy is clearly afraid of the virus itself, so it was coded as fear of AIDS. While death, loss, and suffering are a part of the experience of HIV, they are not unique to HIV and were not, for coding purposes, determined to be relevant to protagonist fears about the disease in and of itself. Therefore, only those fears that related directly to contracting HIV or to social ramifications of HIV infection were coded.

Fear statements were coded based on various types of expressions in the narratives. Where fear statements were explicit, that is, a character states, "I am afraid," coding was relatively straightforward. Likewise, physiological responses such as dry mouth, closed throat, or racing heart were also coded as fear, based on the context of the story. Additionally, such behaviors as backing away from individuals known to have AIDS, avoiding them, or taking extra care around them (e.g., excessive hand washing), were considered to be statements of fear and were coded as such. To ensure the quality of the data and the clarity of the message, where there was content that was not an explicit statement or thought regarding fear, all researchers came to consensus on whether the message was a fear message.

Coding of protagonist fears was based on manifest content and ranged over five broad categories. These categories included instances where books have no fear content at all and instances where the protagonist is manifestly not afraid. Also included in the discussion are situations where the protagonist is manifestly unsure about feeling afraid. Finally, where fear statements are present, they were categorized as either fears for self or fears for other people. The last two categories contain a set of variables grouped into reasonable fears and unreasonable fears. Reasonable fears are those tied to the actual medical risk of contracting the disease, or of experiencing social isolation or other social and/or interpersonal consequences of HIV infection. Unreasonable fears are those tied to situations where there is no risk of infection from HIV, for example, hugging or sitting next to someone who has HIV.

The following discussion examines the coding process for each of these categories in turn.

FEAR CODING PROCEDURES AND EXAMPLES

In all cases, fear messages were coded by first noting whether fear content is present and, if so, the nature of that content. In addition, if a novel contains more than one protagonist, the name of the one expressing the fear message was recorded. Direct quotes were copied and page numbers noted. If there was a fear for self or others present, the reason for that fear was recorded as well, based directly on the content of the fear message, and it was determined whether that fear is reasonable (i.e., based on medically proven risks of contracting the disease) or unreasonable (i.e., not tied to any true risk factors for transmission).

No Fear Content

Several of the books in this body of literature contain no messages regarding HIV-related fear. In some instances, this absence of fear content actually signifies an ignorance (or ignoring) of actual risk factors, as in *Night Kites* when Erick is sleeping with Nikki, who has recently broken up with a drug dealer.[7] AIDS is in Erick's family, but he ignores the risks he is taking with Nikki, despite the fact that he knows her past and he knows that a person can have HIV and not show it. Likewise, Christian in *Rebel without a Clue* is having unprotected sex with a girl who is currently promiscuous and has slept with drug dealers in the past, but he is worried only about his HIV-infected friend's protected sex.[8] In contrast, Anna, who has lost a brother to AIDS, shows no fear of the disease in *What about Anna?*[9] HIV is a presence throughout the book, but Anna is familiar with the risks and knows how to manage them and so experiences no fear.

Manifest Content of No Fear

Many books in this body of literature have no HIV-related fear content. This is to be contrasted with the current discussion, where fear content is manifest, but it is manifestly a *lack* of fear. Sometimes this coding relied on statements that protagonists make (or think), and other times it relied on manifest behaviors that demonstrate a lack of fear. An example of the latter is Michael in *Never Tear Us Apart*,[10] who kisses his HIV-positive uncle on the cheek. He does not say he is not afraid, but he also does not shy away. Likewise, Leyla, upon learning in *The Beat Goes On* that her cousin Emma is HIV positive, "hugged her and held her as tight" as she could.[11] Claire, in *The Deeper, the Bluer*,[12] considers helping women with HIV because her mother is HIV positive, and she has also read quite a bit about it. This evidences a manifest lack of fear of contracting HIV. And Colin, in *Two Weeks with the Queen*,[13] is not afraid of visiting Griff in the hospital because he knows you do not catch AIDS that way.

Sometimes, however, a protagonist will say outright that he or she is not afraid. Jenna, for instance, in *Soul Love*, states, "I know Gabe would never do anything to put me in danger";[14] and Elaine, in *Red Hair Three*, experiences the same confidence that the person she loves is not going to do anything to put her in danger, even though he is HIV positive.[15] Claire, in *What Happened to Lani Garver*, understands that many people are afraid of AIDS, but for her, "talking to someone my own age who knew about anything this serious . . . it gave me a rush."[16]

Not Sure

Emotions are often complicated. One might feel a number of emotions at the same time, even sentiments that conflict, like fear and not being afraid. In these times, it can be difficult to parse out and express a single emotion. This is true in novels as in life. In these cases, a fear message of "not sure" was coded to reflect this internal conflict. Allie, for example, in *Be Still My Heart*, thinks, "I'm not scared. . . . I'm not sure about that. I may be scared."[17] And Karen, in *Until Whatever*, tries to reassure herself she will not get AIDS by sitting at the same table with someone, but then thinks, "I wish I felt as sure about that as I sounded."[18]

Fear for Self

When protagonists express fear that they might possibly contract HIV or suffer other consequences of HIV infection, including social isolation, this was coded as "fear for self." A protagonist might reasonably be afraid of contracting HIV after having had unprotected sex, as is Robin in *Robin's Diary*.[19] Likewise, he or she might be unreasonably afraid to sit next to someone known to be HIV positive, as is Lexi in *The Discovery*.[20]

Fear for Others

When a protagonist expresses fear for someone else, this was coded as "fear for others." The name of the person for whom the protagonist fears was added to the coding. This fear can be directed at someone the protagonist knows who is engaging in risky behaviors, like Kyle who fears for Nelson in *Rainbow Road*.[21] Fear can also be directed toward people with whom the protagonist does not have a direct relationship, as in *Good-Bye Tomorrow*, where Christy is afraid for the girls who kissed Alex, her brother, who is HIV positive.[22]

Reasonable Fear and Unreasonable Fear

The following discussion addresses the particular dimensions of fear messages encountered in this body of novels in terms of whether these messages are based on true risks for contracting the disease. Medical science has demonstrated that HIV is transmissible only three ways: (1) through sex with someone already infected with HIV; (2) through contact with infected blood, most commonly now through sharing needles (e.g., for injecting street drugs or steroids) with someone already infected with HIV; and (3) through vertical transmission from a mother to her infant either in utero or through breast-feeding. Each of these potential causes features an exchange of bodily fluids, but the concentration of HIV in fluids other than blood, semen, or breast milk has been found to be minimal and unlikely to spread the virus. Protagonist fears related to these potential causes of HIV were considered to be reasonable fears.

HIV is only transmissible through the aforementioned means. Because the concentration of HIV in fluids other than blood, semen, or breast milk has been found to be minimal and unlikely to propagate the virus, any other protagonist fear messages related to contracting HIV were considered to be unreasonable because they are not based on true risk factors. These fears range from fears of kissing or sharing food with someone who is HIV positive to simply being in the same room (or town) as someone who is HIV positive, to those fears for which no concrete reason is provided at all.

The following discussion examines individual reason codes for expressed fears in terms of fear for self and fear for others and whether each fear is reasonable.

Positive Test Results

The most immediate reasonable fear related to contracting the disease is a positive result on an HIV test. If someone tests positive for HIV, he or she is at risk of getting AIDS, regardless of how the virus was transmitted. In *Good-Bye Tomorrow*, when Alex receives his test results, his response is a physical fear reaction: "'Does it mean I have AIDS?' My face grew hot just saying the word. I leaned forward in the chair, hands gripping my knees."[23]

In *Playing with Fire*, Sofia is scared for her sister Rosa, who has just disclosed her positive HIV test results: "I do not know what I feel. Maybe tired, sad, and afraid. Or afraid, tired, and sad. . . . For as long as I didn't know, there was a cold lump in my stomach. Now the chill has spread right through my body."[24] In *I Never Got to Say Good-Bye*, Traci is worried for Mark because, "She'd read enough about AIDS to know this was serious."[25]

Often, when a fear is directly related to HIV but with someone who is already known to be HIV positive, this fear was coded under "positive test results." For example, Desi in *Baby Alicia Is Dying* already knows that Alicia is HIV positive, and the fear she experiences for Alicia is HIV specific.[26] This was coded as fear related to positive test results.

Unprotected Sex

Unprotected sex is a significant risk factor for contracting HIV. When a protagonist has had unprotected sex and subsequently worries about contracting the disease, the unprotected sex was considered to be the source of the fear. Sometimes, the fear and the cause are close together in the text, for example in *Push*, when Precious thinks, "Then oh! No! Oh no, I get all squozen inside. Carl fuckes me. I could be done have it."[27] Here, the fear is tied directly to unprotected sex. But in *Robin's Diary*, although Robin and Stone have chosen not to use condoms because she is on the pill, she does not refer directly to this when mentioning her fear: "I'm scared. I'm scared. I'm scared. What if I am? What if I have it? What if Stone gave it to me?"[28]

When fear for others related to unprotected sex was coded, the fear is sometimes based on the actions of the protagonist and sometimes based on the actions of the person for whom the protagonist fears. For example, in *Good-Bye Tomorrow*, one of the protagonists, Alex, is concerned for his girlfriend Shannon because they had unprotected sex before he knew he was HIV positive.[29] He is worried about the possibility that he infected her with HIV. Whereas in *Get It While It's Hot. Or Not*, Megan is worried about her pregnant friend Kit because the father of the baby is known to be a steroid injector and HIV positive.[30]

Multiple Partners

Even when safe sex is practiced, the risk of contracting HIV increases with the number of partners with whom one is sexually active. In *Playing with Fire*, for example, the protagonist Sofia is worried about her sister Rosa's lifestyle because Rosa has had multiple sex partners.[31]

Vertical Transmission

Because vertical transmission of HIV occurs between mother and infant, all fears related to vertical transmission in this set of novels were fears for others. In *Earthshine*, for example, Slim is concerned for her friend's unborn baby sister because his mother is HIV positive: "Oh lord, I think, as my heart comes crashing into my throat. 'The baby. . . . Are you—is she—are they doing okay?'"[32] And in *Push*, Precious is afraid for her toddler son upon learning that she herself is HIV positive.[33]

Intravenous Drug Use

Intravenous drug use is a significant risk factor for HIV transmission. Some young people inject such street drugs as heroin or cocaine, while others inject more "mainstream" drugs like steroids. There is no fear content related to intravenous drug use in this population of books.

Exposure to Blood

While the HIV virus is short-lived outside the body and exposure to blood is a risk that can be managed with simple precautions, fear of contracting HIV through blood exposure is generally considered to be a reasonable fear. Coding in these instances was relatively straightforward. In *Until Whatever*, for example, HIV-positive Connie has just accidentally cut her finger and is bleeding: "Not a lot, just a few drops, but deadly drops," Karen realizes. "'Hand me a Kleenex,' [Connie] says. I don't move."[34] Here fear has immobilized the protagonist. In contrast, Christian, in *Rebel without a Clue*, is very careful about cleaning himself after he has been exposed to the blood of his HIV-positive friend Thomas.[35]

In *Robin's Diary*, Robin is afraid for her uncle after he is exposed to the blood of her HIV-positive boyfriend: "Uncle Mac has Stone's blood down the front of him . . . [Felicia] is afraid about the blood and so am I."[36] And in *Touch of the Clown*, Barbara is scared when her little sister goes running after a ball; she wants to get it herself to avoid Livvy possibly finding an infected drug needle hidden in the bushes.[37]

Sometimes, however, the fear of exposure to blood is considered to be unreasonable. In *Laura Leonora's First Amendment*, for example, Laura is afraid of any blood, including her own uninfected blood, because she has misconceptions about how HIV is transmitted.[38] Her fear is considered in this instance to be unreasonable. Likewise, Clinton, in *Fade to Black*, is hyperbolically afraid of donating blood because, "You don't always know where those needles have been, no matter what they tell you."[39] In fact, needles used for blood donation are used only once and then discarded in specially designed receptacles for biohazardous waste.

Future Sex

The fear of potential future sexual encounters is a common theme running through this set of novels. Some protagonists are afraid they will not be able to make good choices, while others are just afraid of the overall risk of contracting HIV after becoming sexually active. Nico, in *Woman Soldier/La Soldadera*, fantasizes about Reyno, for example, although she knows he has had sex with many girls and that it makes him a risky partner.[40] She worries, "What if she lost control of herself and had sex with him?," while arguing with herself that, "On the other hand, he is handsome."[41] While Debra, in *What You Don't Know Can Kill You*, who has not yet had sex but whose sister is now HIV positive, wonders, "Will I be risking my life too?,"[42] and she states that, "The very thought of sex made her feel sick."[43]

When the protagonist fears for others regarding future sex, that fear may be for the person with whom he or she has a relationship or it may be for the people his or her loved one might infect, either through carelessness or indifference. In *Rainbow Road*, Kyle worries about his flighty best friend Nelson going off with someone they met on their trip, because Nelson is under the influence of drugs and not likely, even in the best of circumstances, to make the healthiest choice.[44] But in *Raging Skies*, Jenny is not worried about her friend Amelia, who is HIV positive, but about Amelia's love interest, Kareem, because, "[Amelia] says that if a person is thoughtless enough to have sex without a condom and take the risk of getting her pregnant, then he deserves the consequences."[45]

Violence

Although HIV-related discrimination and other negative social responses to those infected with HIV have diminished in the three decades since the first diagnosis of AIDS, these problems do still exist.[46] While not directly related to contracting HIV, fears regarding these types of consequences of HIV infection were considered, for the purposes of the project, to be valid HIV-related fears. In *Until Whatever*, Karen holds a party at her house, and only two other people attend, one of whom is her HIV-positive friend Connie, but they are visited by others who are hostile: "A rock lands on the floor," having been tossed through a now broken window; "The truth is, I'm scared," Karen admits.[47]

Discrimination

Discrimination is another social problem related to HIV that was determined to be a reasonable fear. Alex, for example, in *Good-Bye Tomorrow*, is "afraid to think how I'd be treated if it got around about me."[48] These fears are also manifest for others, as in *The Mayday Rampage* when Jess worries about how the town will react to the news that his favorite teacher has a lover who is dying of AIDS: "They'll crucify him. They'll probably burn down his house or something. He'll never get another job in this town."[49] And Alex, in *Good-Bye Tomorrow*, worries about the repercussions of his HIV-positive status with his girlfriend: "If it ever got out that I have the virus, everybody would figure you have it too. No guy would ever come near you."[50]

Social Isolation

Fear of social isolation is a common theme in a number of these novels. Again, this social fear was determined to be reasonable based on continued incidences of stigma that persist even into the present day. In *Chanda's Secrets*, Chanda states,

> A million terrible thoughts fill my head. Are we without friends from this moment on? Cut off? Shunned? Left to live and die alone? I fill with fear. I can't say the problem out loud. I don't want it written down or connected to my family.[51]

Not Knowing What to Do

In the more personal realm, Leyla, in *The Beat Goes On*, worries that she will not know how to help her cousin Emma, who is HIV positive. She is afraid of saying the wrong thing, of acting differently around her when she just wants things to be normal:

> At times, since Emma had told me about the HIV, I'd felt like a little girl plonked in the middle of a totally grown-up situation with no guidebook, no rules, or instructions on how to find my way around. I was scared of making a really big mistake.[52]

Losing Control

In *Chanda's Secrets*, Chanda worries that she will lose control over the situation once it gets out that her mother has died of AIDS: "What if the city finds out? What if they take Soly and Iris away? Would they? Could they? I don't know. . . . Will Mrs. Tafa take over? Will she steal my family?"[53]

Casual Contact

Manifest protagonist fear related to contracting HIV via casual contact is evidenced in a variety of ways in this set of novels. Some protagonists worry that touching someone with HIV might somehow infect them, as in the case of Binti in *The Heaven Shop*, who worries about holding on to the HIV-positive Jeremiah on a bicycle ride to fetch her sister.[54] Likewise Lexi, in *The Discovery*, does not want to sit next to Nancy, who is HIV positive.[55] And Rhan, in *Ran Van: Magic Nation*, who, upon learning that an acquaintance is HIV positive, "pulled away, a knee-jerk of alarm that was so obvious he was embarrassed. . . . But knowing better didn't mean you could stop it."[56]

Other protagonists worry about breathing the same air as a person with HIV, like Jane in *Born Blue*, who states that, "Her AIDS germs was all over the place,"[57] and Clinton in *Fade to*

Black, who says, "I always try not to breathe too much when I'm in class with him."[58]

Fear of contracting HIV through casual contact is not limited to fear for oneself, however. In *A Dream to Cherish*, for example, Cassie is concerned about Tommy, the boy who skates with HIV-positive Arien;[59] and Clinton, in *Fade to Black*, worries about his younger sister visiting Alex's sister because, "we don't know what kind of germs and spores and junk is flying around their house."[60]

Saliva, Tears, Sweat

HIV has never been found to be transmitted through the exchange of bodily fluids other than blood, semen, and breast milk,[61] yet fears of contracting HIV through saliva, tears, and sweat are often expressed by protagonists in this body of literature. These fears were coded individually as fear of tears, fear of kissing, fear of sharing food, fear of nasal mucus, fear of sweat, and fear of saliva, but they are grouped together here under exchange of harmless bodily fluids.

Sarah, for example, in *Rumors and Whispers*, is afraid of kissing David, who is HIV positive,[62] and Traci, in *I Never Got to Say Good-Bye*, fights her fear about Mark using the same dishes she does: "sometimes I won't even pick up Mark's glass. And after he's used a spoon or something, I have to force myself not to go wash it with bleach like our housekeeper does."[63] In *Laura Leonora's First Amendment*, Laura worries about someone with AIDS crying,[64] as does Karen in *Until Whatever*.[65] Cassie, in *A Dream to Cherish*, avoids Arien's sweaty socks,[66] and Clinton, in *Fade to Black*, worries about Alex sneezing.[67]

Lacy, in *My Brother Has AIDS*, is anxious about spreading HIV to others, so she thinks she should not share her food with other people even though she knows AIDS does not spread that way.[68] And in *Good-Bye Tomorrow*, Christy is afraid for the girls Alex kissed at the New Year's party.[69] These were coded as unreasonable fears for others related to sharing food and kissing, respectively.

No Reason Given

Often a fear statement was encountered that had no other context to assist in parsing out that to which the fear was tied.

In each of these cases, the fear was determined unequivocally to be related to HIV (as opposed to death or loss, for example) before being coded. Any time a reason is not provided for a protagonist's HIV-related fear, it was determined to be an unreasonable fear.

Allie, in *Be Still My Heart*, for example, is "worried and scared a lot"[70] because a teacher's spouse has HIV, but no risk factors can be derived from the text. Likewise, Cassie, in *A Dream to Cherish*, is "absolutely terrified of an invisible virus and of the girl who carried it,"[71] but there are no risk factors present that would reasonably incite this fear. Laura, in *Laura Leonora's First Amendment*, is afraid for her family and for the whole seventh grade, but again, no reason is given and no risk factors are present.[72]

FINDINGS

The system described above was used to code each of the books in this set of novels in terms of fears that protagonists experience related to HIV/AIDS and the nature of those fears. The following section presents the findings from this work. A total of 341 messages of fear were discovered and coded, of which 292 indicate fear on the part of the protagonist and the remainder are manifestly "no fear" or "unsure." There are, however, significant outliers that tend to skew the results, so the findings are discussed in terms both of the entire population and of the population without the outliers. Table 3.1 shows the distribution of fear messages, including those books that had no fear content.

Table 3.1. Presence of Fear Content

	Frequency	*Percent*
No content	25	6.8
Not sure	2	0.5
No	47	12.8
Yes, self	205	56
Yes, other	87	23.9
Total	366	100

No Fear Content

Just more than one quarter of the books included in this study, 25 of the 93 titles inclusive (26.1 percent), contain no fear messages. This means that there were no statements regarding fear in the text in these cases.

Manifest Content of No Fear

Direct statements or actions that indicate an actual manifestation of a protagonist's lack of fear regarding particular instances of perceived HIV risk were also coded. Of all the HIV fear–related messages in this set of novels, 47 (12.8 percent) of these messages are statements that indicate a lack of fear.

Not Sure

In only 2 cases (0.6 percent), the protagonist expresses an ambivalence that wavers between being afraid and not being afraid. These instances were coded as "not sure," because the protagonist is manifestly unable to decide, in a given moment, whether he or she is afraid of HIV. These messages are not present in books where HIV was only mentioned in passing.

Yes, Afraid for Self

The majority of fear messages in these novels are HIV-related fears the protagonist has for himself or herself. When examined in terms of all fear messages present, including those messages that indicate no fear, the 205 messages of fear for self constitute 56 percent of the total. When viewed in terms just of those messages of present fear, however, the percentage rises to 70.2 percent. The proportion of fear for self in relation to fear for others, therefore, is higher.

Two outliers skew these results, however. *Fade to Black*,[73] with twenty-four messages of fear, and *Good-Bye Tomorrow*,[74] with fifty-three fear messages, both contain significantly more fear messages than the other books. When the outliers are taken out of the picture, there are only 134 messages of fear for self, which account for 52.3 percent of all manifest fear messages and 64.7 percent of those messages where fear is present.

Yes, Afraid for Others

In those novels where fear content is present, eighty-seven of the fear messages address a protagonist's fears for other people in his or her life. When viewed in terms of all fear messages, this constitutes 23.9 percent and, in terms only of where fear is manifestly present, it is 29.8 percent. When the outliers are taken out of the picture, the percentages of fear for others rise to 28.5 percent and 35.3 percent, respectively.

Reason Codes

Findings connected to reason codes for fear messages are discussed in the following section in order of their frequency of occurrence overall. Results when outliers are removed change the order and frequency, but the findings are presented in terms of all incidences where fear is manifestly present and differences are noted as appropriate. There are 292 manifest instances of protagonist HIV-related fear, and when outliers are removed this number drops sharply to 207. Figures 3.1 and 3.2 illustrate the

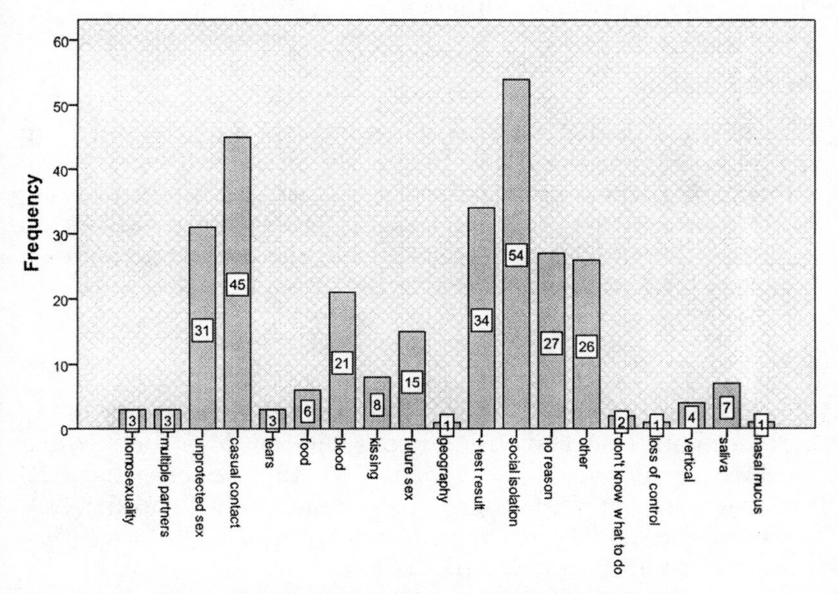

Figure 3.1. Reason for Protagonist Fears, Outliers Included

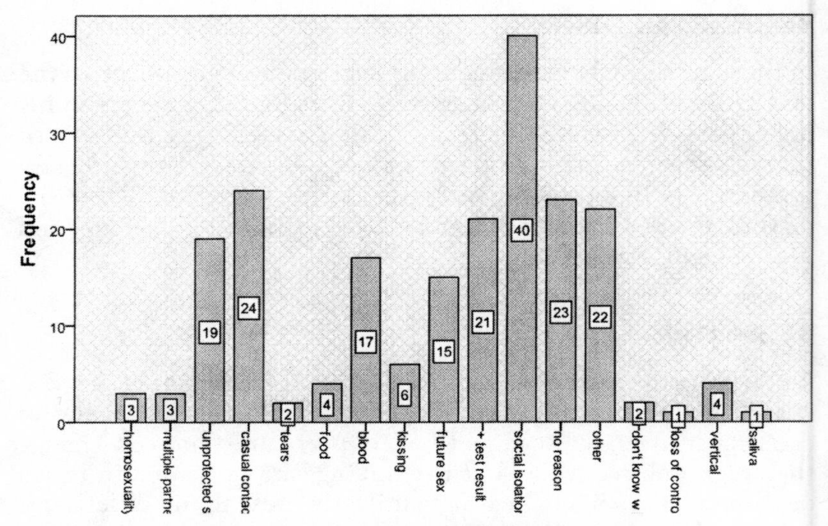

Figure 3.2. Reason for Protagonist Fears, Outliers Removed

distribution of reason codes. The first includes the outliers, and the second removes the outliers from the analysis.

Social Isolation

Fear of social isolation, even when outliers are removed from the analysis, tops the list of frequently mentioned fears. When all instances where protagonists experience fear are considered, 54 (18.5 percent) are related to social isolation. When outliers are removed, the number decreases (40), but the percentage actually increases (19.3 percent) because of the ratio of types of fears.

Casual Contact

Similarly, fear of casual contact falls second in frequency of occurrence both with and without consideration of outliers. When outliers are included in the analysis, 45 (15.4 percent) fear messages are present regarding casual contact. When outliers are removed, the number of fear messages drops to 24, but the difference in percentage is less stark (11.6 percent).

Positive Test Results

Here, the results diverge. Fear of HIV related to positive test results falls next in order of frequency when outliers are included in the calculation, but not when the outliers are removed, although the differences are small. When all messages that are indications of fear present are considered, there are 34 (11.6 percent) that address positive test results. When the outliers are removed, there are 21 (10.1 percent) passages.

Unprotected Sex

Thirty-one (10.6 percent) messages of fear related to unprotected sex are present when all fear messages are taken into account. When outliers are removed, however, this number drops to 19 (9.2 percent).

No Reason Given

Twenty-seven (9.2 percent) of all fear messages that address manifest fears are clearly present as fear messages but are not attached to any specific reason in the text. When outliers are taken out of the picture, this proportion actually increases to 23 (11.1 percent). Note that when outliers are removed, this reason code falls directly after fears related to casual contact.

Harmless Bodily Fluids

For the purpose of presenting findings, all bodily fluids deemed to be harmless are grouped together here, including tears, nasal mucus, sweat, and saliva (this would include, for example, sharing food or dishes and also kissing). Fear statements regarding harmless bodily fluids account for 25 (8.6 percent) statements all together and 13 (6.3 percent) statements when outliers are taken out of the analysis.

Exposure to Blood

Fear related to exposure to blood features in 21 HIV-related fear messages when all positive fear messages are taken into account

(7.2 percent). The proportion rises, however, when outliers are removed (8.2 percent), while the number drops only slightly to 17 fear messages. With outliers out of the picture, fears related to blood exposure fall directly after fears related to unprotected sex.

Future Sex

Fifteen fear messages related to having sex at some point in the future are present whether outliers are considered in the analysis or not. If outliers are dropped, however, the percentage of these messages increases from 5.1 percent to 7.2 percent.

Remaining Individually Coded Fears

Several fears related to HIV are mentioned very infrequently in the novels. All numbers and percentages include outliers, as these are so infrequently mentioned that outliers do not change the results. Fear of vertical transmission is mentioned 4 times (1.4 percent). Fear of multiple partners and of homosexuality each appears 3 times (1 percent). Fear of not knowing what to do is mentioned twice (0.7 percent). Finally, fear of loss of control and of geography are each mentioned once (0.3 percent).

Other Fears

HIV-related fears that did not fall into one of the previously mentioned categories were coded as "other." These fears account for 26 (8.9 percent) messages overall and 22 (10.6 percent) messages when outliers are dropped.

Reasonable Fears and Unreasonable Fears

Statements regarding reasonable fears, those fears related to actual medical risk of contracting HIV even if that risk can be managed, accounted for 165 messages out of all instances where protagonists experience fear in this set of novels (56.5 percent). When outliers are removed from the analysis, the numbers decrease slightly, to 122, but the proportion increases slightly, to 58.9 percent. Statements regarding unreasonable fears, however, account for a significant proportion of the total whether all messages are taken into account (127 messages and 43.5 percent) or whether the outliers are dropped (86 messages and 41.5 percent).

DISCUSSION/CONCLUSIONS

The question examined in this chapter is, What are the fears of protagonists regarding HIV? Specific fears are discussed in terms of how they manifest and why, and findings are presented in an effort to answer that question. This section provides a discussion of the implications of the findings and provides additional pertinent information not already addressed in the coverage of the content analysis.

Unreasonable fears are significantly overrepresented in this set of novels, even when mitigating factors are taken into account. A mitigating factor, for example, would be if someone experiences an unreasonable fear and then manages it and does not act on the fear. If we assume that messages about fear provide information about the risks related to HIV disease, then this body of literature is not yet properly meeting a crucial information need of young people related to HIV and its transmission. Unreasonable fear messages can convey the idea that HIV is far more dangerous than it actually is, perpetuating erroneous beliefs and ignoring true risk.

The complete lack of fear messages related to intravenous drug use, for example, ignores this very real risk, one of the main vectors of HIV transmission in young people. Also, in a few instances significant risk factors are present, but there are no corresponding fear messages regarding these risks. For example, in *Night Kites*, Erick is sleeping with a girl who he knows was recently sexually active with a drug dealer, but he expresses no fear related to this or even caution.[75] In *Zach at Risk*, Zach has a neighbor who is gruesomely dying of AIDS. Moreover, Zach has been molested by the owner of the shop where he works part-time. Yet when he goes to get tested for HIV, he displays no fear.[76] And Brian, in *Never Tear Us Apart*, is extremely promiscuous, but neither he nor any of his friends or conquests ever express worry over this.[77] There are clearly HIV-related information needs that are not yet being met through this body of literature.

This does not provide a complete picture of the status of the literature, however. In some instances, the lack of expressed fear can be considered an indication that HIV/AIDS has been simply disregarded as a risk, as in the case of *Zach at Risk*, where even in the face of a person dying of AIDS and Zach's own molestation, it just simply does not register as worthy of fear.[78] *Night Kites* provides another example, demonstrating the invisibility of HIV, which is played out both in the lack of attention to the risks and in the apparent lack of awareness that risk is present even when the disease is not visible.[79]

In other novels, however, the lack of fear messages can be an indication that while risks for contracting HIV exist, these risks can be managed. In *The Deeper, the Bluer*, for example, Claire does not express fear, but it is because she has a full awareness of how HIV is transmitted and she knows how to take care of herself and her mother, who is HIV positive.[80] In *What Happened to Lani Garver*[81] and *What about Anna?*,[82] HIV plays a minor role in the story, but it is present in a matter-of-fact way that does not directly address specific risk factors but that does treat HIV as something that need not be feared in casual situations. In essence, fear does not come up in these novels because there is simply no reason for fear to surface, even though HIV is present.

Another item not fully captured in the findings is the way that fears are addressed once they have been expressed. One can either manage the fear and come to an understanding and acceptance of what are true risks and what are not, or one can succumb to those fears and perpetuate them. In *What You Don't Know Can Kill You*, for instance, Ellen is HIV positive and has fears regarding her disease; however, she manages these fears by reaching out for support within her family, among her friends, and in a support group for people who are diagnosed with HIV.[83] She thus learns to take control of her disease and her life, and she matures and becomes more independent as a result. In contrast, her boyfriend Jack is so consumed with fear that he commits suicide. Anne Wingate, in *Sixteen and Dying*, is also so overcome by fear related to her HIV-positive status that she essentially shuts down.[84] She provides a telling example of the consequences of letting fear take control.

In addition to protagonists who are themselves infected with HIV and experience fear, there are also those who are not HIV positive who experience fears related to contracting the disease. Some manage these fears effectively and some do not. The unnamed narrator in *Now That I've Found You*, for example, has a momentary lapse of reason when he learns that his girlfriend is HIV positive and he remembers that he has already kissed her. However, he talks himself down from this, reminding himself that HIV is not transmitted through kissing.[85] Likewise, Binti, in *The Heaven Shop*, briefly experiences fear when invited to ride a bicycle with Jeremiah, who is HIV positive, but she is reminded by Jeremiah that you cannot contract AIDS just by touching someone.[86] She knows this, but the gentle reminder is enough to help her manage her fear until it is all but forgotten. In *A Dream to Cherish*, however, Cassie repeatedly lets her admittedly unreasonable fears keep her from being with and helping her friend who is HIV positive.[87] While mitigating messages are overtly present, the fact that Cassie continues to let her fears guide her behavior is telling. There are also some instances that go almost completely unchallenged, like the school nurse in *Until Whatever* who refuses to treat Connie because Connie is HIV positive.[88] Another example of someone who should know better but goes essentially unchallenged is the hospital nurse at Arien's bedside in *A Dream to Cherish*.[89] The nurse wears a face mask connected to oxygen and is covered head to toe to avoid touching or even breathing the same air as the girl who has AIDS. These sorts of unchallenged messages are certainly not going to meet the information needs of young adults who may be fearful about how HIV is transmitted.

Another place where the content analysis requires further elucidation is when there is a manifest lack of fear. Sometimes this overt lack of fear is related to ignorance or a willful ignoring of the risks. Nelson, in *Rainbow Road*, manifestly does not worry about becoming infected with HIV while trying to find a partner during a cross-country road trip.[90] He disregards the fact that he is often high on drugs when searching out partners and is thus very likely to make poor decisions.

Messages of overt lack of fear can also be very positive messages, however. In *Two Weeks with the Queen*, for example, Colin visits the HIV-positive friend of a new friend in the hospital.[91] Colin also shares food with Griff, feeling safe in the knowledge that "you could only catch it off stuff from inside the body, blood and stuff like that."[92] It is treated as a matter of course and no precautions need to be taken. This is a positive message about the true risks of HIV. Another positive message that takes a different tack is in *Ran Van: Magic Nation*, when Lee, who is HIV positive, has been shot.[93] There is blood everywhere, posing a significant risk, but Rhan is unafraid and also deeply aware. He finds a place on Lee's body where there is no blood and places his hand there. He thus protects himself while offering the best kind of support that can be offered to a person who is dying in front of him—being there and being unafraid.

Another message that manifest no fear content can convey is that of support of the person with HIV and a level of commitment to taking care of that person. Leyla, for example, in *The Beat Goes On*, demonstrates both her lack of fear and her commitment to her cousin by hugging her as tightly as she can after learning that Emma is HIV positive.[94] Claire, in *The Deeper, the Bluer*, shows no fear of her mother's HIV, offering her verbal encouragement, saying, "You're strong, Mama,"[95] and considering a career in helping other women who have HIV because she now knows so much about it and is unafraid.

Often, messages of no fear are like a shout of defiance both against HIV and against the fear it can generate, as in *Chanda's Secrets* when Chanda says, "I don't care what people think anymore."[96] Claire, in *What Happened to Lani Garver*, actually gets a rush from knowing people who understand what she has been through as a person in remission from leukemia.[97] Shannon, in *Good-Bye Tomorrow*, plans for several friends to escort Alex, who is HIV positive, to school on his first day back, to "show everyone we're not afraid."[98] Sarah, in *Rumors and Whispers*, assures her mother, somewhat testily, that, "There's no evidence that I could possibly catch AIDS from Mr. Hill."[99]

Fade to Black provides a special case worth considering in this discussion.[100] This novel is an outlier as far as the number and types of fear messages present, but Clinton, the one expressing most of the fears, is clearly an unreliable narrator. Fear messages are thus overtly present and ubiquitous, but they are spoken in Clinton's voice and often either directly preceded or directly followed by messages from people who are more knowledgeable and reasoned about the risks. This actually serves to render the meaning of the book the direct opposite of the meaning of the content that was coded for the purposes of this project.

While there are instances like those previously mentioned that help provide a more nuanced picture of the risks associated with HIV/AIDS, this body of literature still shows some significant gaps in pertinent information. It is hoped that these gaps will be filled more effectively for young people as the pandemic continues and with it research on managing and living with HIV.

NOTES

1. Alex Flinn, *Fade to Black* (New York: HarperTempest, 2005), 17.
2. Alex Sanchez, *Rainbow Boys* (New York: Simon & Schuster, 2001).
3. Flinn, *Fade to Black*.
4. Alice Hoffman, *At Risk* (New York: Putnam, 1988).
5. Deborah Davis, *My Brother Has AIDS* (New York: Jean Karl/Atheneum, 1994), 71.
6. Davis, *My Brother Has AIDS*, 148.
7. M. E. Kerr, *Night Kites* (New York: HarperTrophy, 1986).
8. Holly Uyemoto, *Rebel without a Clue* (New York: Crown Publishers, 1989).
9. Jan Simoen, *What about Anna?*, trans. from Dutch by John Nieuwenhuizen (New York: Walker & Company, 2002).
10. Quinn Brockton, *Never Tear Us Apart*, A "Queer as Folk" Novel (New York: Pocket Books/Simon & Schuster, Inc., 2003).
11. Adele Minchin, *The Beat Goes On* (New York: Simon & Schuster, 2004), 15.
12. Barbara Field, *The Deeper, the Bluer* (Lincoln, NE: iUniverse.com, 2000).
13. Morris Gleitzman, *Two Weeks with the Queen* (New York: Putnam, 1991).
14. Lynda Waterhouse, *Soul Love* (London: Piccadilly Press, 2004).
15. Charlotte St. John, *Red Hair Three* (New York: Fawcett Juniper, 1992).
16. Carol Plum-Ucci, *What Happened to Lani Garver* (Orlando, FL: Harcourt, 2002), 39.
17. Patricia Hermes, *Be Still My Heart* (New York: G. P. Putnam's Sons, 1989), 121.
18. Martha Humphreys, *Until Whatever* (New York: Clarion Books, 1991), 16.
19. Judith Pinsker, *Robin's Diary* (Radnor, PA: ABC Daytime Press/Chilton Book Company, 1995).

20. Judy Baer, *The Discovery*, Cedar River Daydreams, No. 20 (Minneapolis: Bethany House, 1993).
21. Alex Sanchez, *Rainbow Road* (New York: Simon & Schuster, 2005).
22. Gloria D. Miklowitz, *Good-Bye Tomorrow* (New York: Delacorte Press, 1987).
23. Miklowitz, *Good-Bye Tomorrow*, 57.
24. Henning Mankell, *Playing with Fire*, trans. from Swedish by Anna Paterson (Crows Nest, NSW, Australia: Allen & Unwin, 2002), 122.
25. Alida E. Young, *I Never Got to Say Good-Bye* (Worthington, OH: Willowisp Press, 1988), 129.
26. Lurlene McDaniel, *Baby Alicia Is Dying* (New York: Bantam, 1993).
27. Sapphire, *Push* (New York: Vintage Contemporaries, 1996), 85.
28. Pinsker, *Robin's Diary*, 88.
29. Miklowitz, *Good-Bye Tomorrow*.
30. Valerie Hobbs, *Get It While It's Hot. Or Not* (New York: Richard Jackson/Orchard, 1996).
31. Mankell, *Playing with Fire*.
32. Theresa Nelson, *Earthshine* (New York: Orchard Books, 1994), 164.
33. Sapphire, *Push*.
34. Humphreys, *Until Whatever*, 56.
35. Uyemoto, *Rebel without a Clue*.
36. Pinsker, *Robin's Diary*, 155.
37. Glen Huser, *Touch of the Clown* (Buffalo, NY: Groundwood, 1999).
38. Miriam Cohen, *Laura Leonora's First Amendment* (New York: Lodestar Books/Dutton, 1990).
39. Flinn, *Fade to Black*, 161–62.
40. Irene Beltrán Hernández, *Woman Soldier/La Soldadera* (Waco, TX: Blue Rose Books, 1998).
41. Hernández, *Woman Soldier/La Soldadera*, 159.
42. Fran Arrick, *What You Don't Know Can Kill You* (New York: Bantam Books, 1992), 116.
43. Arrick, *What You Don't Know Can Kill You*, 118.
44. Sanchez, *Rainbow Road*.
45. Nancy Mitchell, *Raging Skies*, Changing Earth Trilogy, Book Two (Fremont, CA: Lightstream Publications, 1999), 170.
46. Gregory Herek, John Capitanio, and Keith Widaman, "Stigma, Social Risk, and Health Policy: Public Attitudes toward HIV Surveillance Policies and the Social Construction of Illness," *Health Psychology* 22, no. 5 (2002): 533–40.
47. Humphreys, *Until Whatever*, 130.

48. Miklowitz, *Good-Bye Tomorrow*, 88.
49. Clayton Bess, *The Mayday Rampage* (Sacramento, CA: Lookout Press, 1993), 177.
50. Miklowitz, *Good-Bye Tomorrow*, 100.
51. Allan Stratton, *Chanda's Secrets* (New York: Annick Press, 2004), 183.
52. Minchin, *The Beat Goes On, 99.*
53. Stratton, *Chanda's Secrets*, 144.
54. Deborah Ellis, *The Heaven Shop* (Allston, MA: Fitzhenry & Whiteside, 2004).
55. Baer, *The Discovery.*
56. Diana Wieler, *Ran Van: Magic Nation* (Buffalo, NY: Groundwood Books/Douglas & McIntyre, 1997), 189.
57. Han Nolan, *Born Blue* (New York: Harcourt, 2001), 247.
58. Flinn, *Fade to Black*, 5.
59. Angela Elwell Hunt, *A Dream to Cherish*, Cassie Perkins Series, No. 4 (Lincoln, NE: Authors Guild Backinprint.com Edition/iUniverse .com, 1992).
60. Flinn, *Fade to Black*, 5.
61. Centers for Disease Control and Prevention (CDC), "HIV and Its Transmission," 1999 (last reviewed by the CDC on March 8, 2007). Available at www.cdc.gov/hiv/resources/factsheets/transmission.htm (18 November 2009).
62. Marilyn Levy, *Rumors and Whispers* (New York: Fawcett Juniper/ Ballantine Books, 1990).
63. Young, *I Never Got to Say Good-Bye*, 154.
64. Cohen, *Laura Leonora's First Amendment.*
65. Humphreys, *Until Whatever.*
66. Hunt, *A Dream to Cherish.*
67. Flinn, *Fade to Black.*
68. Davis, *My Brother Has AIDS.*
69. Miklowitz, *Good-Bye Tomorrow.*
70. Hermes, *Be Still My Heart*, 36.
71. Hunt, *A Dream to Cherish*, 137.
72. Cohen, *Laura Leonora's First Amendment.*
73. Flinn, *Fade to Black.*
74. Miklowitz, *Good-Bye Tomorrow.*
75. Kerr, *Night Kites.*
76. Pamela Shepherd, *Zach at Risk* (New York: Alice Street Editions/ Haworth Press, 2004).
77. Brockton, *Never Tear Us Apart.*
78. Shepherd, *Zach at Risk.*
79. Kerr, *Night Kites.*
80. Field, *The Deeper, the Bluer.*

81. Plum-Ucci, *What Happened to Lani Garver.*
82. Simoen, *What about Anna?*
83. Arrick, *What You Don't Know Can Kill You.*
84. Lurlene McDaniel, *Sixteen and Dying* (One Last Wish) (New York: Bantam, 1992).
85. Rex Harley, *Now That I've Found You* (Llandysul, Ceredigion, Wales: Pont Books/Gomer Press, 2003).
86. Ellis, *The Heaven Shop.*
87. Hunt, *A Dream to Cherish.*
88. Humphreys, *Until Whatever.*
89. Hunt, *A Dream to Cherish.*
90. Sanchez, *Rainbow Road.*
91. Gleitzman, *Two Weeks with the Queen.*
92. Gleitzman, *Two Weeks with the Queen*, 118.
93. Wieler, *Ran Van: Magic Nation.*
94. Minchin, *The Beat Goes On.*
95. Field, *The Deeper, the Bluer*, 143.
96. Stratton, *Chanda's Secrets*, 191.
97. Plum-Ucci, *What Happened to Lani Garver.*
98. Miklowitz, *Good-Bye Tomorrow*, 148.
99. Levy, *Rumors and Whispers*, 150.
100. Flinn, *Fade to Black.*

4

How Controllable Is HIV/AIDS?

> "I'll probably get it eventually anyway. If I do, I'll go on meds. *You* do it."
>
> —Alex Sanchez, *Rainbow High*[1]

When the virus that has come to be known as human immunodeficiency virus (HIV) was first being studied, many people equated HIV infection to a death sentence. Later, as the disease became better understood and increasingly efficacious treatments were developed, a transition occurred in which those who are infected are increasingly referred to as living with HIV rather than dying of AIDS.

While it is true that both a cure for HIV and the development of a vaccine remain elusive, current treatments for HIV are extending life for many. For example, where medical care is available, the incidence of vertical transmission (mother to child) has been greatly reduced. Likewise, treatments have made it possible for many HIV-infected babies to survive, and many are now among the young adult population. In recent news a new approach to vaccine development resulted in a small but statistically significant reduction in infection. Scientists were not able to explain how the vaccine, RV 144, works, as it does not appear to produce antibodies in the way most vaccines do, nor did the vaccine affect the viral load of people who received it but ended up infected with HIV anyway.[2] Other analyses of this trial have called into question whether the outcome described was actually due to statistical chance, rather than treatment.[3] While the findings from this study are important, they do not signal that scientists are anywhere near producing a vaccine that could be made commercially available. Further, there is the problem that this news may be misinterpreted by some, resulting in an increase in risky behavior.[4] Dr. Julio Montaner, president of the International AIDS Society and director of the B. C. Centre for Excellence in HIV/AIDS, said, "Even if a future vaccine is effective enough to pass regulatory approval, it would have to be used along with other tools such as public education and increased HIV screening."[5]

This change in the perception of HIV has both positive and negative aspects. While the introduction of highly active antiretroviral therapy (HAART) has had a positive effect in terms of extending life for many, this may be leading to an attitude of complacency about infection. There are in fact people who actively seek infection with HIV (dubbed "bug chasers") and others who "help" these individuals by offering to infect them (referred to as "gift givers"). It appears that bug chasers seek out infection for a number of reasons, including the idea that the "virus just isn't a big deal anymore," that infection is inevitable anyway, and that being infected will take the worry out of sex and restore a sense of freedom.[6]

In fact, while current treatments are extending lives, this does not mean that the quality of life for those with HIV infections is comparable to that of noninfected individuals. There are HIV-infected individuals who are less helped than others by the available treatments. These include people who are not able to tolerate the treatments or who are unable to comply with them, people whose infection has already advanced to AIDS by the time they learn they are infected, and people who are infected with a strain of HIV that is resistant to one or more of the available drugs.[7] The Centers for Disease Control and Prevention (CDC) estimates that one-fourth of those infected with HIV are unaware of their health status.[8]

While improvements to the regimens required to maintain health for the HIV infected have in some cases become less onerous, treatment can still be difficult to adhere to, and there are a number of serious side effects related to anti-HIV medications, for example, liver damage, diabetes, abnormal fat distribution, lactic acidosis, nerve problems, pancreatitis, and more.[9] HIV/AIDS is not currently curable and can still be disabling.

Early detection and treatment are key to extending life, but scientists are still working on understanding the progression of the disease, which varies from person to person. The period between initial infection and the development of AIDS appears to be impacted by many factors. Some factors that appear to hasten the progression of HIV to AIDS are "older age, infection with more than one type of HIV, poor nutrition, and severe stress."[10] Factors that appear to lengthen life include medical care, good nutrition, and other general health practices.[11]

Another consideration is the cost of treatment. A study conducted by a team of researchers from the Partners AIDS Research Center/Massachusetts General Hospital Cornell, Johns Hopkins University School of Medicine, Harvard School of Public Health, Harvard Medical School, and Boston University School of Public Health concluded that while HIV treatment can extend life up to twenty-four years, the cost of monthly care for an individual averages about $2,100 per month, or a lifetime cost of $618,900.[12] More than 70 percent of this cost is for medication. Estimated costs go up to $4,700 a month when HIV is not detected until it has progressed to AIDS, as treatment involves more hospital care.[13]

These costs naturally bring up issues of medical insurance and government funding for care, as the cost of care affects its availability for many. The least expensive option is prevention. The projected treatment expense that could be avoided through prevention is estimated at $303,100 per person.[14]

ARE HIV/AIDS CHARACTERS DEPICTED AS LIVING WITH HIV OR DYING OF AIDS?

The research questions addressed in this chapter focus on the presence and type of control messages found in these young adult novels and the fate of the characters with HIV/AIDS. These two factors—indication that HIV can be controlled and the fate of the infected—combine to provide a picture of whether these novels depict infection with HIV as a death sentence or as an illness that can be managed.

Noting the presence or absence of control messages is important, because in the early years of publication of this body of literature the idea that HIV infection is essentially a death sentence was pervasive, although messages of control were beginning to be seen in these books.[15]

CODING CONTROL MESSAGES

The first level of coding for control consists of three categories that look at whether the individual books make statements about the ability to control the disease or not. The first category is the absence of any content related to the question of whether the disease can be controlled. The second category is the presence of control statements that are immediately qualified by a conflicting statement, and the third is the presence of manifest content clearly indicating that there is some method for controlling the disease.

No Content

Sometimes a lack of control content is a result of the fact that a particular book is not primarily about HIV/AIDS, for example *The Car*.[16] There are also books with subplots that involve HIV/AIDS that make no statement about control. An interesting example of this is *Under the Big Sky*, in which Travis learns that his ex-boyfriend is HIV positive and that he and his current boyfriend, Cash, have to wait out testing to see if Travis is HIV positive, too.[17]

There are also books that do not talk about control but do talk about HIV infection as fatal. For example, in *Be Still My Heart* there are no statements of control, and while the HIV/AIDS character is healthy and strong, his wife confides to the protagonist, "He's dying Allie. And I'm missing him already."[18] Indications that the progression of HIV cannot be controlled are not coded, as this is considered the baseline assumption in these books. The fate of HIV-infected characters works to provide another view of whether HIV/AIDS is manageable.

Qualified Statements of Control

It also happens that although a narrative may make many statements about the availability of treatments and other types of control, these are not always efficacious as far as the HIV/AIDS character is concerned or are contradicted by other content in the story. In *Changing Jamie,* Billy the bug chaser states, "We're going to get it eventually, and it's not a big deal anymore, anyway. There are drugs for it now."[19] However, the protagonist, Jamie, equates AIDS with death throughout the novel, and when Billy succeeds in getting infected he learns that the regimen for maintaining his health is expensive and difficult to tolerate.

In *Sixteen and Dying,* there are many references to AZT as treatment; however, the protagonist, Anne, avoids treatment because she does not want to experience the side effects.[20] It is made clear in the narrative that there is no cure for AIDS and that Anne will die (see the title). It is only a question of how long it will take. In Anne's case, it takes less than a year.

Like *Sixteen and Dying,* there are many titles that foreshadow for the reader that the story is about loss and death whether there are other clues on the book jacket or cover that the story involves a character who is HIV positive or who has AIDS. These titles include *I Never Got to Say Good-Bye,*[21] *Losing David,*[22] *What You Don't Know Can Kill You,*[23] *The Silent Killer,*[24] *When Heroes Die,*[25] *Until Whatever,*[26] *Baby Alicia Is Dying,*[27] *Good-Bye Tomorrow,*[28] *Something Terrible Happened,*[29] and *Unfinished Dreams.*[30] In these cases, the fate of the character is prescribed before the reading even starts and overrides the idea that control of HIV infection is possible.

Control statements also come into play when characters have to face the fact that someone they know has HIV/AIDS. A common response in these narratives is to assure the HIV-infected character that control is possible. Some of these statements are more convincing than others. For example, in *Rebel without a Clue* Christian tells his friend Thomas, "They come closer every day to finding a cure," but then he confesses that, "I told him, not knowing who 'they' were and not certain why I was saying it. I had no idea whether or not the truth was coming into play at all, my current events knowledge was so pitiable."[31]

Control Is Possible

Manifest indications of control do appear in these books, revealing the presence of the idea that HIV can be managed. Examples include *Soul Love*, in which the reader is told, "It can be controlled by medication but there is no cure";[32] *Rainbow High*, where Nelson muses, "I'll probably get it eventually anyway. If I do, I'll go on meds"[33] and later pronounces, "No one dies of AIDS anymore except perhaps in Africa";[34] and *What You Don't Know Can Kill You*, where HIV-infected Ellen asserts there is no need to worry about her, saying, "If I get sick, then I'll have to be treated."[35]

CODING REASONS WHY CONTROL IS POSSIBLE

In addition to coding the presence and absence of control statements, the control statements themselves were analyzed for the type of control identified as possible. The types of statements may vary in their strength and, as noted above, some are more convincing than others. For example, the idea that there are treatments that can help is a stronger statement of control than is "think positively" or that there is hope for a future cure. The categories of control coded from these books are presented and discussed in the following section.

Treatment Is Available

One of the most concrete signs that HIV/AIDS is controllable is the fact that treatments are available now to help manage the disease and extend life. The code "treatment is available" was used when HIV/AIDS characters talk about treatment regimens and when the availability of treatments is discussed. For example, in *The Discovery*, Nancy provides this update on her condition: "My doctor and I are considering AZT, an AIDS treatment drug. There is hope that, while a cure for AIDS may not be found for a long time, we can learn to deal with it as a chronic illness. New facts are being learned every day."[36]

In *University Hospital: Heart Trauma*, the following information about treatment and avoiding HIV infection is shared: "nowadays, with AZT and other drugs, AIDS doesn't have to be passed from mother to baby."[37]

Maintaining or Adopting Healthy Habits

This code reflects the CDC guidelines for maintaining health for those infected with HIV, which includes such advice as "eat healthy foods," "exercise regularly," "get enough sleep," and "take time to relax."[38] Demonstrations of this advice being given or that HIV/AIDS characters are taking this advice were coded as "maintaining or adopting healthy habits." For example, in *The Arizona Kid*, Billy says about Luke, "He looks like an ad for vitamins," and Uncle Wes responds, "He goes to his yoga class, his acupuncturist, his nutritionist, his counselor, and he takes his AZT."[39]

In *Something Terrible Happened*, the following recommendations for caring for Gillian's HIV-infected mother are offered: "We don't want her to worry. We have to make sure she eats right, takes vitamins, gets plenty of rest. . . . Proper nutrition is the main thing. . . . Don't overlook ol-time [sic] cures either."[40] Similarly, in *Playing with Fire*, Sofia writes in her diary, "He [Dr. Nkeka] explained that it is a serious illness, but gave her some hope of living for a long time if she looks after herself. She must eat lots of vegetables, think happy thoughts, and carry on leading her life the way she always has, from first thing in the morning until late at night."[41]

Hope of New Treatments

The idea that HIV/AIDS will be increasingly controllable is found in statements characters make about new drugs being developed and the promise that new treatments are imminent. Examples of this coding include such statements as, "A new drug that shows promising results for Wasting Syndrome is approved by the FDA. It is called Clarythromycin. A similar drug, Azithromysin, is slated for approval soon," in *The Mayday Rampage*,[42] and "'The government is pouring millions of dollars into research,' Traci went on. 'We keep reading about new drugs to help,'" in *I Never Got to Say Good-Bye*.[43]

Hope of a Future Cure

The code "hope of a future cure" reflects the idea that medical science will one day be able to cure HIV infection. For example, in *The Discovery*, the reader is told, "There are people working day and night looking for a cure. You can't give up hope."[44] Similar statements are expressed in *Real Heroes*: "With the research that's going on now, there's the possibility that with proper medical treatment, people may be able to live a normal lifetime with HIV and never develop AIDS."[45]

Healthy Now

"Healthy now" coding records messages given to HIV-infected characters that they should focus on the idea that they are healthy now and that health can be maintained. In *Chanda's Secrets*, Nurse Viser says to Esther, "The good news is, your health is excellent and you may be able to get treatment before you're sick."[46] In *Rainbow High*, Nelson clarifies Jeremy's health status saying, "He has HIV. . . . That doesn't mean he's sick. He's healthier than I am."[47] Likewise in *The Beat Goes On*, "Emma still looked and acted so normal, and although there were a few changes, like the food and tablets I knew she had to take, her life went on pretty much as usual."[48]

Education about HIV/AIDS

Since the *Surgeon General's Report on Acquired Immune Deficiency Syndrome*, released in 1986, control of HIV infection through education has been a focus of many government agencies and private organizations.[49] Coding of statements about the use of educational interventions to control the spread of HIV reflect this effort. Examples of statements coded in this way include Jeremiah's explanation of his efforts to educate others in *The Heaven Shop*: "Condoms, brochures about HIV, blood-testing kits. I'm a peer counselor. I travel on my bike and talk to other young people—well, any people, actually—about protecting against AIDS, and how to take care of themselves if they have AIDS."[50] Another example is the assertion in *The Discovery* that, "Education is one way to stop the virus from spreading."[51]

Thinking Positively and/or Faith

The CDC guidelines for staying healthy for those infected with HIV also suggest that, "Many people find that meditation or prayer, along with exercise and rest, help them cope with the stress of having HIV or AIDS."[52] While some may consider faith and thinking positively to be a weaker control message than the availability of treatments, it is a concept that is presented in this body of literature as a way to control HIV/AIDS. In *I Never Got to Say Good-Bye*, HIV-infected Mark is told, "you have to have a positive attitude,"[53] and in *Something Terrible Happened*, the following advice is given: "The main thing is trusting in God."[54]

Social Support

"Social support" as a way of managing HIV/AIDS infection conveys the help that family and friends can provide and the benefits of continuing to function within various social support mechanisms. In *My Brother Has AIDS*, regardless of the misgivings Jack's family may have about his illness, he is taken into the home and assured that he will be okay because, "You're here and we're helping you."[55]

In *What You Don't Know Can Kill You*, an excellent example is provided of a young woman coping well with her diagnosis and living with HIV. This is possible at least in part because, "Ellen spent as much time as she could with [her friend] Annie. . . . Annie Adler was Ellen's treatment."[56] Likewise, in *The Heaven Shop*, the reader is told that, "People, even in Malawi, can live for a long time with HIV if they have a good diet and people who love them."[57]

Others Living Successfully with HIV

Sometimes in these stories the idea that a person can successfully live with HIV is demonstrated by pointing to an example of someone who embodies this goal through their lifestyle, appearance, or longevity. In *University Hospital: Heart Trauma*, the reader is told, "I met a guy in Paris who's been HIV positive for like ten years and he has no symptoms . . . the scumbag's fine."[58]

Another example is Jon Hanley in *Robin's Diary*, who is seen repeatedly in the background of the story and who is presented as a role model for the newly diagnosed Stone. The reader learns that Jon Hanley was, "diagnosed *nine years ago*, and is going strong."[59] A similarly long-lived character from real life, the French singer Mano Solo, makes multiple appearances in *What about Anna?*, in which he reminds his audience that he is still alive.[60] In *The Arizona Kid*, HIV-infected Luke is also living successfully with

HIV/AIDS. "He's everybody's role model, because when he had pneumonia, nobody was sicker than he was. And now look at him. So people say, 'If Luke can do it, I can do it.'"[61]

Limited Access to Medical Care

This code captures the idea that treatment is available for HIV infection but not for everyone. In books set in the developed world, the main issues are often the cost of medical care and lack of insurance. In settings outside of the developed world, drugs may be too expensive or just unavailable. For example in *Strays Like Us*, which takes place in the United States, the HIV-infected father of the protagonist's friend is housed in the attic and his presence kept secret.[62] There is no insurance, and his care is left to his family and neighbor, who do the best they can to assist him. Similarly, in *The Mayday Rampage*, Jess and Molly marry so that she can share his health insurance and thereby afford the treatment she needs.[63]

Examples of coding limited access to medical care for books that take place in the developing world include *The Heaven Shop*, where Jeremiah says, "It's true that there's no cure. . . . People in rich countries have AIDS drugs that help a lot, but few people here can afford them. But that doesn't mean we are helpless."[64] In *Playing with Fire*, the reader is told that, "Deolinda had heard that in other countries, there were people with plenty of money who could buy expensive medicines. These medicines, and having the best doctors and a really good life, meant that they could live for as long as practically anybody else. That certainly was not true for Rosa."[65]

Control Indicated but No Reason Given

In some of the narratives the idea that it is possible to live with HIV infection is asserted, but no reason is given for why this is so. In *Tommy Stands Alone*, Frank relates a conversation about his brother in which his mother says, "He's going to be fine, but they found out he's HIV positive,"[66] and in *Diving for the Moon* the reader is told, "It's better these days. Josh may live for years."[67] These statements are reassuring, but they are not backed up with evidence for why there is no reason to worry.

Other

The "other" category is designed to catch instances of control that do not fit into the predefined categories previously discussed. The books that discuss other kinds of control offer a range of reasons. In *The Arizona Kid* we learn that Billy's friend's father has a plan to "cure AIDS and cancer and all that stuff." The plan, however, is the annihilation of the human species. "He says that's the upside of thermonuclear war."[68]

At the other end of the spectrum, both *Baby Alicia Is Dying* and *I Never Got to Say Good-Bye* suggest that love is the way to control HIV infection. In *Baby Alicia Is Dying*, the protagonist is told that, "Sometimes a whopping dose of love can be more effective than all the hospital care in the world."[69] Likewise, in *I Never Got to Say Good-Bye*, the protagonist is advised that the best way to help her uncle is to "just give him lots of love."[70] *The Mayday Rampage* offers a more practical approach, suggesting that distributing condoms and clean needles is a way to control HIV infection.[71]

FINDINGS ON CONTROL MESSAGES

All of the books identified for this study were read and coded as previously described to determine if they contain messages that HIV is controllable and to record the reason given as to why this is so. What follows is a presentation of the findings on control and reason statements for this body of literature.

Indications That HIV Can Be Controlled

The majority of the books included in this study (59 or 63.4 percent) contain some indication that control of HIV/AIDS is achievable for infected individuals. Indications that control of HIV is possible begin as early as the publication of *Night Kites*, although the statement, "There were still plenty of AIDS victims who hadn't died yet" is not particularly confidence building.[72] Of these 59 titles, 5 books (or 5.3 percent of 93 titles) offer only a qualified statement about the possibility of control.

Eighteen books (19.3 percent of 93 titles) include both clear statements that control is possible as well as qualified statements about control. The ratio of qualified statements as compared to clear statements of control in books that contain both tends to be low. Only 5 out of these 18 books (27.7 percent) have 2 qualified statements of control. The other 13 (72.2 percent) contain only 1 qualified statement of control. The number of positive statements in these 18 books range from 1 to 28. The average number of positive statements is 6.2.

There are 36 books (38.7 percent of the 93 coded) that make only positive clear statements about the possibility of living a full life after HIV infection. On the other hand, 34 (36.5 percent) of the 93 books examined contain no statements about control.

Reasons Given in Control Statements

The most frequent reason cited for why it is possible to live with HIV infection is the message that medical treatments are available to help. Statements of this type represent 95 (36.5 percent) of the reasons why control is possible offered in these texts. The next largest category is "maintaining or adopting healthy habits," which accounts for 34 (13.1 percent) of the reasons given. There were 28 (10.8 percent) "hope of a future cure" statements and 20 (7.7 percent) statements each for the categories pointing to the power of thinking positively (or having faith) and statements that there are examples of other people living successfully with HIV infection. All other reason codes that accompanied an indication that control is possible represented less than 7 percent of the reasons given. Figure 4.1 provides a full breakdown of the frequencies.

When the reason codes are analyzed for how they relate to clear statements of control and qualified statements of control, fewer reason codes are represented when control statements are qualified. The main reasons offered in a qualified way are (in order of frequency): treatments are available (12 statements or 36.4 percent of qualified statements); hope of new treatments (5 statements, 15.2 percent of qualified statements); limited access to medical care (5 statements, 15.2 percent of qualified statements); hope of a future cure (3 statements, 9.1 percent of qualified statements); healthy now (2 statements, 6.1 percent of qualified statements); others are living successfully with HIV (2 statements, 6.1 percent of qualified statements); other (2 statements, 6.1 percent

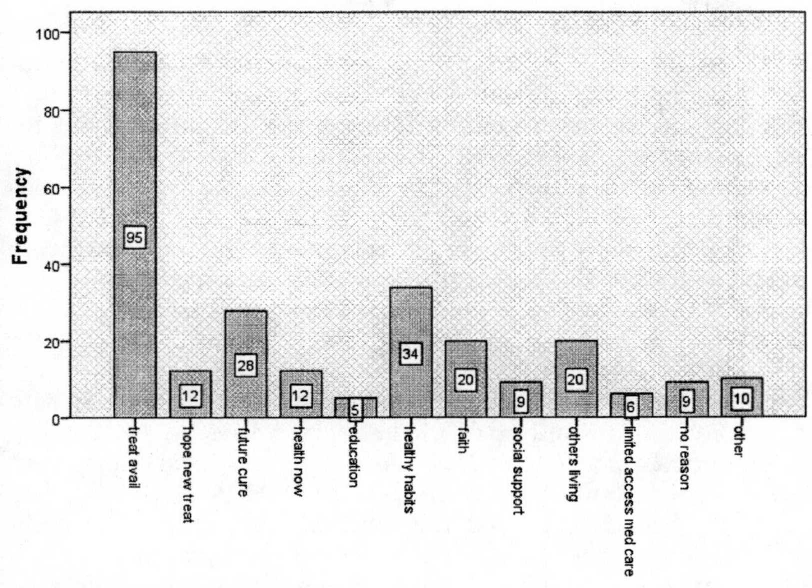

Figure 4.1. Reason Codes

of qualified statements); social support (1 statement, 3 percent of qualified statements); and no reason (1 statement, 3 percent of qualified statements).

Messages about Fate

Another way of considering whether these books communicate the message that HIV infection is fatal or that it is possible to manage HIV infection and continue to live a full life is to discover what happens to characters who have HIV/AIDS. Whether these characters live or die, or are depicted as dying, as well as the extent to which the fate of these characters is unknown, provides information about what the outcome is for people infected with HIV and to what extent living with HIV is possible.

The fate of HIV/AIDS characters in these novels was described in the coding in four ways. In each case, as with the other coding performed for this content analysis, manifest content was used to determine outcomes. The categories used include: text does not say, lives, dying or death imminent, and dies.

Text Does Not Say

The first category, "text does not say," applies when the narrative provides no indication of the fate of a character. Sometimes this happens because an HIV/AIDS character is a minor character in the story who appears for a time but is not central enough to the action for his or her fate to be tracked. There are several types of characters who fall into this category for different reasons. One factor is that there are many HIV characters who are countable but who are not important to the main action of the story. For many of these characters there is no reason within the narrative to track their fate, as they are not relevant to or do not remain relevant to the plot line.

The development and importance of these characters, who are of concern for only part of the story, varies. In *Notes from a Spinning Planet: Papua New Guinea*, several characters share their stories about how they contracted HIV; however, once they have been interviewed, they become part of the background as Maddie and her journalist aunt continue their investigation of HIV infection in New Guinea so they can write a magazine article.[73] Jeremy, one of Nelson's previous love interests, comes up briefly in *Rainbow Road*, but he is relegated to the past as Nelson's head is quickly turned by the boys he meets on a cross-country road trip.[74]

As noted in chapter 2, there are many characters in these books who are only relevant in that they are the source of infection for HIV/AIDS characters who are more central to the story. Examples include the blood donor in *At Risk*,[75] the rapist in *Now That I've Found You*,[76] and Emma's one-night stand in *The Beat Goes On*.[77] There are also many other minor HIV/AIDS characters who are barely mentioned at all, such as the street people encountered in *Random Acts of Senseless Violence*,[78] the assembly speaker brought in to talk to students about HIV/AIDS in *Overnight Sensation*,[79] and people in line at the hospital to receive care in *The Heaven Shop*.[80]

Lives

For HIV/AIDS characters who remain a part of the main story, the code "lives" is used if there is no indication that they are dying or have died within the narrative. Interestingly, in one story,

The Last Vampire, the HIV-infected character not only lives but is cured of his illness.[81] Seymour is cured by the vampire, Alisa Pern, who shares her super immunity by giving him enough of her blood to cure him but not enough to turn him into a vampire. She does this so that he can live to write the story of her long life.

Dying or Death Imminent

There are many cases where it is made clear that the HIV/AIDS character is going to die. For example, in *Night Kites*, Erick's brother Pete tells him, "It's okay. . . . We can talk about my dying."[82] In *Until Whatever*, Karen says, "Whatever, I sense the future. Connie's in the hospital now. . . . She'll come out, but eventually she'll go in again. And again. And again. And finally, one time, that'll be it."[83] A third example is found in *When Love Comes to Town*, when Neil visits his friend Daphne (also known as Eddie) and remarks, "He's going to die, isn't he, Jesus?"[84]

Dies

The category "dies" was recorded as a character's fate when the text makes it clear that this is the outcome. For example, in *Baby Alicia Is Dying*, the fate of the baby born to a drug-using mother is captured in the short phrase, "She's gone."[85] Likewise, in *Two Weeks with the Queen*, the reader learns that Griff, who has been in the hospital with AIDS, "died this morning."[86] In many of the books characters talk of people from the past who had AIDS and died from it, and these expressions of fate were coded as "dies." For example, in *Earthshine*, the reader learns that Mr. Dodd, husband to the HIV-infected and pregnant Angelina, "died a few months ago."[87]

FINDINGS FOR FATE

In this set of books there are 376 HIV/AIDS characters who are described as distinct individuals. The most frequent category coded for these characters is "dies" (160 instances or 42.6 percent of 376). An additional 9 characters (2.4 percent) are dying by the time the narrative ends. The second largest category for fate is

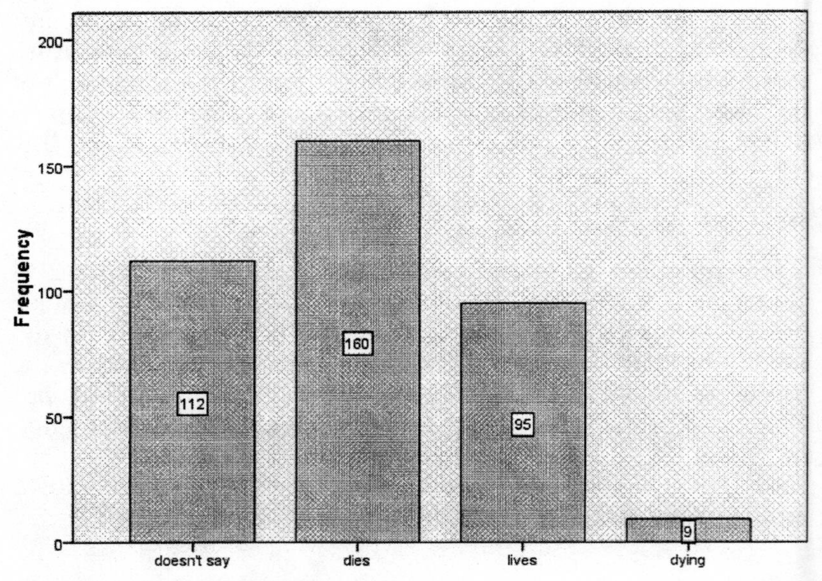

Figure 4.2. Fate of HIV/AIDS Characters

"text does not say," which represents 112 (29.8 percent) of the characters in these books. Only about a quarter (95 or 25.3 percent) of the HIV/AIDS characters in these stories live. Figure 4.2 displays these frequencies.

Who Dies of AIDS?

An analysis of the fate of HIV/AIDS characters based on their relationship to the protagonist reveals that the largest category of characters who die or are clearly dying in these books are characters with whom the protagonist has no relationship (74 characters or 43.7 percent of dying or dead characters). The next largest category is "extended family" (30 characters or 17.7 percent of dying or dead characters). "Friend's family/friend" accounts for 13 characters (7.6 percent of dying or dead characters). The rest of the dying and dead characters are sprinkled across the remaining relationship categories.

Interestingly, an analysis of who "lives" reveals that the largest relationship category with this fate is also people with whom the protagonist has no direct relationship (28 or 29.4 percent of HIV/AIDS characters who live); however, the relationship "friend" comes in a close second at 21 living characters (22.1 percent of all characters who live). Further, friends with HIV/AIDS represent 65.6 percent of these characters. Another interesting finding is that when the protagonist is the person with HIV/AIDS, 7 out of the 9 live (77.7 percent).

When fate is considered on the basis of age, characters in the young adult age range (eleven to nineteen years) fare better than any other age group. Among characters whose age is manifestly given in the narrative as in this age range, 35 (64.8 percent of 54 characters) live, 0 are dying, 12 (22.2 percent) die, and in 7 cases (13 percent) the text does not say what happened to them. Likewise, children birth to age four also tend to fare better than other groups. Of the 18 characters who unambiguously fall in this category, 9 (50 percent) live, 1 (5.6 percent) is dying, 6 (33.3 percent) die, and for 2 (11.1 percent) the text does not provide an outcome.

In comparison, characters who clearly fall into the category of adult (ages twenty-six to sixty-four) are more likely to die. Of the 146 characters in this category, 21 (14.4 percent) live, 2 (1.4 percent) are dying, 75 (51.4 percent) die, and for 48 (32.9 percent) the text does not reveal their fate.

Characters who are not well enough developed for age to be even guessed at also tend to die. Of the 67 characters for whom no age data was given, 6 (9 percent) live, 1 (1.5 percent) is dying, 37 (55.2 percent) die, and for 23 (34.3 percent) no fate data are provided.

When fate is considered on the basis of gender, female characters have a proportionately better chance of living than males. Among female characters, 36 (32.1 percent) live, 1 (0.9 percent) is dying, 43 (38.4 percent) die, and for 32 (28.6 percent) the text does not reveal their fate. Among male characters, 56 (25.7 percent) live, 8 (3.7 percent) are dying, 94 (43.1 percent) die, and for 60 (27.5 percent) the text does not say what happened to them. Among characters whose gender could not be determined, 3 (6.5 percent) live, 0 were coded as dying, 23 (50 percent) die, and for 20 (43.5 percent) their fate is unknown.

SUMMARY AND CONCLUSIONS

This chapter looks at data related to statements that HIV infection can be controlled and at the fate of HIV/AIDS characters in this set of books. This was done to determine if this body of literature presents HIV as a condition that can be managed or equates HIV infection with a death sentence. As noted earlier in this chapter, the CDC reports that being under the care of a doctor and following such general health practices as eating well, exercising, and avoiding stress are associated with living longer with HIV.[88]

These factors are reflected in the control messages found in these books. The idea that treatment is available and that maintaining or adopting healthy habits is key to living with HIV are realistic messages that control is possible. While these are the kinds of messages most frequently provided in these books, they represent less than half of the control messages expressed in these texts.

While some of the remaining control messages have some validity, for example, education is extremely important to HIV prevention, there were only 5 messages about prevention across 93 books. This is surprising, as the need for education as perhaps the most efficacious way to avoid HIV infection was first called for in 1986, by Surgeon General Koop, and remains the focus of many efforts to stop the spread of HIV. While the idea that education can help stop the spread of infection is not often offered in control statements, school assemblies on the topic of HIV/AIDS occur in *Be Still My Heart*,[89] *The Discovery*,[90] *Overnight Sensation*,[91] and *Touch of the Clown*.[92] In *The Last Safe Place on Earth*, a speaker comes to school, but almost no one attends the meeting.[93]

Other examples of how education about HIV prevention is approached in these stories include the story of *The Mayday Rampage*, which centers on the efforts of two students to educate their peers about HIV/AIDS.[94] Likewise, in *Rumors and Whispers*, parent meetings, which are also attended by some students, provide a forum for discussing the facts about HIV infection and representing the mind-set of some who remain skeptical about this information.[95]

The remaining control messages, often meant to "buck up" HIV characters or those who care about them, are relatively weak messages that offer hope rather than an objective sense that an individual can manage HIV infection and maintain a high quality of life. After "treatment is available" and "maintain or adopt healthy habits," the next most frequent category of control is "no reason given." While the hope of new treatments and the hope of a future cure are worth considering, they are balanced against the fact that a vaccine and cure for HIV remain elusive, even given recent breakthroughs.[96] Improvements in treatment have been made and people are living longer with HIV, but the treatments are still onerous and they do not work for everyone. Infection with HIV continues to be a real risk for young adults.

Other messages like "thinking positive and/or faith" and "social support" offer ideas that may have some palliative effect, but they are not sufficient in and of themselves to provide a fully convincing argument that HIV is a manageable condition. When HIV characters are asked to focus on the fact that they are "healthy now" or that "others are living successfully with HIV," only a very limited sense of control is asserted. The progression of HIV in the body is not fully understood, and one person doing well may not be indicative of outcomes for others. Furthermore, the example that others are living with HIV implies that if others can, so can anyone who is HIV infected; however, not everyone can tolerate the treatments that are currently available, and the prognosis for an individual may depend upon how far the infection has already progressed by the time he or she is diagnosed as HIV positive. The slogan, "Be there for the cure" is meant to be encouraging. So is the idea that HIV-infected people need to "fight." On the flip side, there may be a hidden message that those who are HIV infected are themselves at fault if they are unable to survive until medical science comes up with a cure. The representation of HIV-infected individuals has political and social implications that have been analyzed by Susan Sontag[97] and expressed in critical analysis of adult fiction that deals with HIV/AIDS.[98]

Control as an Issue of Access to Medical Treatment

The idea that treatment is available is the most convincing of the control statements, but it is countered at times by the lack of available medical care, medical insurance, or financial assets. While the coding captured some direct statements about issues of access, in many cases depiction of issues of medical care were not couched in terms of control statements. Rather, the settings and circumstances presented in the books influence the extent to which issues of securing medical care are part of the story being told. For example, depictions of the state of medical care in narratives set in Africa and New Guinea describe hospitals as overcrowded and as places where the HIV infected go to die. There are depictions of community clinics and health care workers who assist people with HIV/AIDS, but these are also balanced with the realities of the limited availability of medicines for most people in these circumstances and the reliance of some characters on traditional medical practices that people believe in but that are not cures or even treatments for AIDS and that, often, serve to spread rather than halt the disease.

In some of the books set in the United States the issues of the cost of medical care are included in the story. For example, in *Strays Like Us*, the HIV/AIDS character is tended to by the neighbor, who does her best but who is ill equipped to meet his medical needs.[99] In *My Brother Has AIDS*[100] and *I Never Got to Say Good-Bye*,[101] the HIV/AIDS characters' families have to shoulder the cost of treatment, and in *The Tragedy of Miss Geneva Flowers*,[102] the HIV/AIDS character is trying to save up for the end-stage care he knows he will eventually need.

The relationship between employment and medical insurance is also addressed in some of these stories. In *Something Terrible Happened*[103] and *The Mayday Rampage*,[104] HIV/AIDS characters lose their health insurance when they are forced to quit their jobs. Also, in *The Mayday Rampage* Molly marries Jess to be insured and get much-needed treatment. In *Night Kites*, Erick's brother Pete barters his resignation for medical insurance knowing that his employer wants him to resign.[105]

Quality of Life

An issue related to control is what it takes to maintain health in the face of HIV/AIDS. Many of these titles make it clear that while treatments are available, they can also be difficult to live with. For example, in *The Tragedy of Miss Geneva Flowers*, Chloe is constantly swallowing pills and suffering side effects to maintain health for as long as he can.[106] In *Changing Jamie*, Billy, a bug chaser, cannot wait to be infected with HIV.[107] Once he achieves his goal, however, he quickly learns that having HIV is not as glamorous as he thought it would be. He has no money for treatment, and treatment is not as simple as he imagined. In *The Eagle Kite,*[108] *Born Blue,*[109] *My Brother Has AIDS,*[110] and *Zach at Risk,*[111] although the HIV/AIDS characters have their medication, they are clearly dying and experience a low quality of life.

Fate

The relative ability to live with HIV/AIDS is also demonstrated in the fate of HIV-infected characters in these stories. Unfortunately, there is a high level of unknown outcome for many of these characters. This, combined with the high proportion of characters who die or are dying, tends to paint a picture of survivability that is vague but leaning away from the idea that one can manage HIV for an extended period of time.

On the other hand, where young adult characters are depicted as having HIV/AIDS, the outcomes presented are more positive. Youth who were infected through vertical transmission are shown to have survived to young adulthood and remain healthy. This accurately reflects the impact of improved treatment on the survivability of these young people. Characters who are friends of the protagonist and protagonists who are infected with HIV are more likely to live than any other age group presented in this literature. This may reinforce the belief in the infallibility of youth in the face of danger or the fact that they have been diagnosed early and have the advantage of medical treatments that were not available to adults at the time of their diagnosis.

In contrast, adults who are HIV positive in these stories are more likely than young people to die. There is only one HIV/AIDS character in the ninety-three books analyzed who might be in the senior age range, but because the age of this character was not explicitly stated he was coded as "adult/senior." The limited number of seniors infected with HIV in these books does not reflect a general absence of senior-aged characters. There are many seniors portrayed that have a place in the lives of young adult protagonists. The fact that seniors are not portrayed as having HIV/AIDS in these stories may signal that people infected with HIV do not survive to see old age or that seniors are not considered to be at risk of HIV infection.

In terms of gender, females have greater survivability than males in these stories, which may be a remnant of the idea that HIV/AIDS is an issue for adult males only. This finding was reported in the first content analysis performed on these works reported in 1998.[112] The movement in these works to include more HIV/AIDS characters in the young adult age range and more female characters who have HIV/AIDS is a positive one in terms of providing narratives that allow young people to see themselves in these stories.

NOTES

1. Alex Sanchez, *Rainbow High* (New York: Simon Pulse, 2003), 14.
2. Donald G. McNeil, "For the First Time, a Vaccine Protects Some from AIDS; Thailand Trials of RV 144 Show Promise, Delighting but Mystifying Scientists," *International Herald Tribune*, September 25, 2009, 1.
3. Donald G. McNeil, "More Doubts Cast on AIDS Study; Debate over Vaccine Trial Held in Thailand Gets Increasingly Complicated," *International Herald Tribune*, October 22, 2009, Leisure, 3.
4. Tu Thanh Ha, "A Huge Boost in the Battle for HIV Vaccine," *Globe and Mail*, September 25, 2009, International News, A3. Elizabeth Pisani, "This Is the Worst Kind of Good News," *Times* (London), September 25, 2009, Editorial, 32.
5. Ha, "A Huge Boost in the Battle for HIV Vaccine," A3.
6. Gregory A. Freeman, "In Search of Death," *Rolling Stone*, January 23, 2003, para. 4. Available at www.rollingstone.com/news/story/5939950/bug_chasers (3 September 2009).
7. Gary Taubes, "Who Still Dies of AIDS and Why," *New York Magazine*, June 8, 2008. Available at http://nymag.com/health/bestdoctors/2008/47569/ (3 September 2009).
8. Jonathan Weil, "Researchers Project Lifetime Cost and Life Expectancy for Current HIV Care in the United States," November 1, 2006. Available at http://weill.cornell.edu/news/releases/wcmc/wcmc_2006/11_01a_06.shtml (18 November 2009).
9. United States Department of Health and Human Services, "Side Effects of AntiHIV Medications," October 2005. Available at www.aidsinfo.nih.gov/contentfiles/sideeffectantihivmeds_cbrochure_en.pdf (3 September 2009). United States Department of Health and Human Services, "HIV and Its Treatment: What You Should Know," December 2008. Available at http://aidsinfo.nih.gov/contentfiles/HIVandItsTreatment_cbrochure_en.pdf (3 September 2009).

10. Centers for Disease Control and Prevention (CDC), "Living with HIV/AIDS," 2007. Available at www.cdc.gov/hiv/resources/brochures/print/livingwithhiv.htm (9 September 2009).

11. Centers for Disease Control and Prevention, "Living with HIV/AIDS."

12. Weil, "Researchers Project Lifetime Cost," 2006.

13. Daniel DeNoon, "Got HIV? Lifetime Cost: $618,900," 2006. Available at www.cbsnews.com/stories/2006/11/02/health/webmd/main2146532.shtml (18 November 2009).

14. Weil, "Researchers Project Lifetime Cost," 2006.

15. Melissa Gross, "What Do Young Adult Novels Say about HIV/AIDS?" *Library Quarterly* 68, no.1 (1998): 1–32.

16. Gary Paulsen, *The Car* (Orlando, FL: Harcourt Brace & Company, 1994).

17. S. Bryan Gonzales, *Under the Big Sky* (Bloomington, IN: AuthorHouse, 2006).

18. Patricia Hermes, *Be Still My Heart* (New York: G. P. Putnam's Sons, 1989), 91.

19. Dakota Chase, *Changing Jamie* (Round Rock, TX: Prizm Books/Torquere Press, 2008), 79.

20. Lurlene McDaniel, *Sixteen and Dying* (One Last Wish) (New York: Bantam, 1992).

21. Alida E. Young, *I Never Got to Say Good-Bye* (Worthington, OH: Willowisp Press, 1988).

22. Elizabeth Benning, *Losing David* (New York: Harper Paperbacks, 1994).

23. Fran Arrick, *What You Don't Know Can Kill You* (New York: Bantam Books, 1992).

24. Barbara Chase, *The Silent Killer* (Kingston, Jamaica: Ian Randle Publishers, 2005).

25. Penny Raife Durant, *When Heroes Die* (New York: Atheneum, 1992).

26. Martha Humphreys, *Until Whatever* (New York: Clarion Books, 1991).

27. Lurlene McDaniel, *Baby Alicia Is Dying* (New York: Bantam, 1993).

28. Gloria D. Miklowitz, *Good-Bye Tomorrow* (New York: Delacorte Press, 1987).

29. Barbara Ann Porte, *Something Terrible Happened* (New York: Orchard Books, 1994).

30. Jane Breskin Zalben, *Unfinished Dreams* (New York: Simon & Schuster Books for Young Readers, 1996).

31. Holly Uyemoto, *Rebel without a Clue* (New York: Crown Publishers, 1989), 21.

32. Lynda Waterhouse, *Soul Love* (London: Piccadilly Press, 2004), 179.

33. Sanchez, *Rainbow High*, 14.

34. Sanchez, *Rainbow High*, 49.

35. Arrick, *What You Don't Know Can Kill You*, 153.

36. Judy Baer, *The Discovery*, Cedar River Daydreams, No. 20 (Minneapolis: Bethany House, 1993), 126.

37. Cherie Bennett and Jeff Gottesfeld, *University Hospital: Heart Trauma*, Book Four (New York: Berkley Jam Books, 2000), 46.

38. Centers for Disease Control and Prevention, "Living with HIV/AIDS."

39. Ron Koertge, *The Arizona Kid* (Boston: Little, Brown, 1988), 72.

40. Porte, *Something Terrible Happened*, 28–29.

41. Henning Mankell, *Playing with Fire*, trans. Anna Paterson (Crows Nest, NSW, Australia: Allen & Unwin, 2002), 122.

42. Clayton Bess, *The Mayday Rampage* (Sacramento, CA: Lookout Press, 1993), 197.

43. Young, *I Never Got to Say Good-Bye*, 62.

44. Baer, *The Discovery*, 61.

45. Marilyn Kaye, *Real Heroes* (New York: Harcourt Brace Jovanovich, 1993), 41.

46. Allan Stratton, *Chanda's Secrets* (New York: Annick Press, 2004), 191.

47. Sanchez, *Rainbow High*, 135.

48. Adele Minchin, *The Beat Goes On* (New York: Simon & Schuster, 2004), 118.

49. C. Everett Koop, *Surgeon General's Report on Acquired Immune Deficiency Syndrome* (Washington, D.C.: U.S. Department of Health and Human Services, 1986).

50. Deborah Ellis, *The Heaven Shop* (Allston, MA: Fitzhenry & Whiteside, 2004), 112.

51. Baer, *The Discovery*, 94.

52. Centers for Disease Control and Prevention, "Living with HIV/AIDS."

53. Young, *I Never Got to Say Good-Bye*, 149.

54. Porte, *Something Terrible Happened*, 29.

55. Deborah Davis, *My Brother Has AIDS* (New York: Jean Karl/Atheneum, 1994), 127.

56. Arrick, *What You Don't Know Can Kill You*, 90.

57. Ellis, *The Heaven Shop*, 140.

58. Bennett and Gottesfeld, *University Hospital: Heart Trauma*, 61.

59. Judith Pinsker, *Robin's Diary* (Radnor, PA: ABC Daytime Press/Chilton Book Company, 1995), 158.

60. Jan Simoen, *What about Anna?*, trans. from Dutch by John Nieuwenhuizen (New York: Walker & Company, 2002).
61. Koertge, *The Arizona Kid*, 72.
62. Richard Peck, *Strays Like Us* (New York: Puffin Books, 1998).
63. Bess, *The Mayday Rampage.*
64. Ellis, *The Heaven Shop*, 113.
65. Mankell, *Playing with Fire*, 129.
66. Gloria Velásquez, *Tommy Stands Alone* (Houston, TX: Piñata Books/Arte Público Press, 1995), 75.
67. Lee F. Bantle, *Diving for the Moon* (New York: Macmillan Books for Young Readers, 1995), 110.
68. Koertge, *The Arizona Kid*, 52.
69. McDaniel, *Baby Alicia Is Dying*, 53.
70. Young, *I Never Got to Say Good-Bye*, 117.
71. Bess, *The Mayday Rampage.*
72. M. E. Kerr, *Night Kites* (New York: HarperTrophy, 1986), 130.
73. Melody Carlson, *Notes from a Spinning Planet: Papua New Guinea* (Colorado Springs, CO: WaterBrook Press/Random House, 2007).
74. Alex Sanchez, *Rainbow Road* (New York: Simon & Schuster, 2005).
75. Alice Hoffman, *At Risk* (New York: Putnam, 1988).
76. Rex Harley, *Now That I've Found You* (Llandysul, Ceredigion, Wales: Pont Books/Gomer Press, 2003).
77. Minchin, *The Beat Goes On.*
78. Jack Womack, *Random Acts of Senseless Violence* (New York: Atlantic Monthly Press, 1994).
79. Scott Johnson, *Overnight Sensation* (New York: Atheneum, 1994).
80. Ellis, *The Heaven Shop.*
81. Christopher Pike, *The Last Vampire* (New York: Archway Paperbacks, 1994).
82. Kerr, *Night Kites*, 179.
83. Humphreys, *Until Whatever*, 147.
84. Tom Lennon, *When Love Comes to Town* (Dublin: O'Brien Press, 1993), 156.
85. McDaniel, *Baby Alicia Is Dying*, 159.
86. Morris Gleitzman, *Two Weeks with the Queen* (New York: Putnam, 1991), 131.
87. Theresa Nelson, *Earthshine* (New York: Orchard Books, 1994), 36.
88. Centers for Disease Control and Prevention, "Living with HIV/AIDS."
89. Hermes, *Be Still My Heart.*
90. Baer, *The Discovery.*
91. Johnson, *Overnight Sensation.*

92. Glen Huser, *Touch of the Clown* (Buffalo, NY: Groundwood, 1999).

93. Richard Peck, *The Last Safe Place on Earth* (New York: Delacorte Press, 1995).

94. Bess, *The Mayday Rampage.*

95. Marilyn Levy, *Rumors and Whispers* (New York: Fawcett Juniper/Ballantine Books, 1990).

96. McNeil, "For the First Time, a Vaccine Protects Some from AIDS," 1.

97. Susan Sontag, *Illness as Metaphor* and *AIDS and Its Metaphors* (New York: Doubleday, 1990).

98. Lawrence Howe, "Review: Critical Anthologies of the Plague Years: Responding to AIDS Literature," *Contemporary Literature* 35, no. 2 (1994): 395–96.

99. Peck, *Strays Like Us.*

100. Davis, *My Brother Has AIDS.*

101. Young, *I Never Got to Say Good-Bye.*

102. Joe Babcock, *The Tragedy of Miss Geneva Flowers* (New York: Carroll & Graf Publishers, 2005).

103. Porte, *Something Terrible Happened.*

104. Bess, *The Mayday Rampage.*

105. Kerr, *Night Kites.*

106. Babcock, *The Tragedy of Miss Geneva Flowers.*

107. Chase, *Changing Jamie.*

108. Paula Fox, *The Eagle Kite* (New York: Orchard Books, 1995).

109. Han Nolan, *Born Blue* (New York: Harcourt, 2001).

110. Davis, *My Brother Has AIDS.*

111. Pamela Shepherd, *Zach at Risk* (New York: Alice Street Editions/Haworth Press, 2004).

112. Gross, "What Do Young Adult Novels Say about HIV/AIDS?"

5

Young Adult Novels with HIV/AIDS Content as a Body of Literature

The purpose of this content analysis is to identify the types of messages about HIV/AIDS that young adults will find in works of fiction. This work was guided by the following five research questions:

1. Which characters have HIV/AIDS in these novels?
2. What is their relationship to the protagonist?
3. How did they contract the disease?
4. What fears, if any, does the protagonist have about contracting HIV/AIDS?
5. What is the fate of HIV/AIDS characters?

This chapter summarizes the points made in previous chapters concerning how young adult novels present information about HIV/AIDS in relation to the research questions posed. It provides a generalized discussion of the strengths and weakness of this subgenre of young adult literature and answers the overarching question, If all that young adult readers knew about HIV/AIDS was the result of reading fiction, what would they know about the epidemic, how the disease is transmitted, and the level of risk HIV/AIDS poses for them personally?

WHICH CHARACTERS HAVE HIV/AIDS IN THESE NOVELS?

The identification of who has HIV/AIDS in these books is important because the characters presented with HIV/AIDS provide one picture of who is at risk of infection. The premise is that when HIV/AIDS characters have a strong relationship to the protagonist, this makes the presence of HIV/AIDS more personal and the risk and consequences of infection more real. For example, when characters who have HIV/AIDS tend to be people with whom the protagonist has no direct relationship, the risk of HIV/AIDS also seems remote. On the other hand, when HIV/AIDS characters are people close to the protagonist and are people the protagonist cares about, the ways that young adults can be affected by the epidemic is demonstrated. This is, of course, most personal when the young adult protagonist is the character infected with HIV.

Information about who has HIV is also conveyed when the age and gender of HIV/AIDS characters are considered. When HIV/AIDS characters are mainly adults, or when HIV/AIDS characters are not well enough defined for age to be determined, the risk of HIV infection may seem remote and be interpreted as an adult problem or the problem of people not associated with young adults. When HIV/AIDS characters depicted are age peers to young adult readers, the idea that young adults are at risk of HIV infection becomes part of the story. Likewise, gender is important for what it conveys about risk and the presence of both male and female HIV/AIDS characters helps to make this point.

Overall, the body of literature analyzed in this study is not yet doing all it might to demonstrate that youth and people they care about are at risk for HIV infection. Most of the people who have HIV/AIDS in these books have little to no relationship to the protagonist. There are only nine protagonists who themselves are HIV positive, and these instances are spread out over the publication period. There is no indication of a trend toward seeing more protagonists who themselves are HIV positive. Likewise, friends and family of the protagonist are depicted as people who have HIV/AIDS, but the numbers are small. There is a propensity for HIV/AIDS characters to be male, although more female characters are appearing in these books. Two groups not represented in these narratives are senior citizens and lesbians.

In terms of the use of background characters—both those that are countable and "uncountable"—there is a distinct difference in presentation between books set in and outside of the developed world. Books set in Africa and Papua New Guinea tend to provide a more visceral sense of the damage the HIV epidemic is wreaking on the populace. The evidence of the destructiveness of HIV is palpable in the vast graveyards, lines of people waiting for treatment, and overcrowded hospitals. While books set in developed countries tend to use statistics to make the point that HIV is a huge problem, the framing of the problem in this way has a remote feel, as the information exists outside of the protagonist's personal life. Thus the human loss that those numbers signify is hard to grasp and also represents someone else's problem. There are many books set in the developed world that focus on main characters only and do not attempt to make statements about the prevalence of HIV infection. While statistics may not have the ability to personalize the problem, the absence of any indication of the impact of HIV/AIDS may reify the mistaken belief of some that HIV/AIDS is no longer a pervasive problem in developed countries.

HOW DID THEY CONTRACT HIV?

This research question assesses how HIV/AIDS characters become infected and the extent to which the reasons given represent real risk factors for young adults. As noted earlier, there are a limited number of ways that HIV is spread. Infection is possible through sexual contact and infected blood, and HIV can also be transmitted from mother to child. Advances in understanding HIV have increased knowledge about how to prevent infection. For example, knowledge of the possibility of transmission through infected blood and blood products has led to the use of universal precautions in handling exposure to blood and the screening of the blood supply. Universal precautions involve the use of "protective barriers such as gloves, gowns, aprons, masks, or protective eyewear, which can reduce the risk of exposure of the health care worker's skin or mucous membranes to potentially infective materials."[1] It is also known that the use of clean needles by intravenous drug users is necessary to stem infection.

Likewise, the sterilization or disposal of equipment that is in contact with blood, for example that used in medical practice and tattooing, increases the safety of these procedures.

Infection rates for the transmission of HIV from mother to child have been greatly impacted by medical interventions. Pregnant women who are identified as HIV positive and who are under the care of a doctor can do much to protect their children from vertical transmission.

In terms of transmission through sexual contact, abstinence, monogamy, and the consistent use of male and female condoms are all ways to limit the possibility of infection. One of the most important means of controlling potential infection is for people to know their HIV status through testing. "Positive prevention" refers to the need for knowledge and support for people who are HIV positive to protect their own health and the health of others.[2] For example, a mother who is unaware that she is HIV positive has a smaller chance of being able to protect her child or extend her own life.

In this content analysis, messages about how HIV/AIDS characters became infected were recorded and analyzed to determine whether they represent real risks that young adults face. The coding category with the largest frequency is "unknown." This lack of information can somewhat be explained, as many of the characters have no direct relationship to the protagonist; however, this leaves an information gap regarding what the risks of infection are and how relevant they are to the lives of young adults. In contrast, the prevalence of heterosexual and homosexual sex as modes of transmission for HIV provides meaningful information that is useful to young adult readers.

The presence of relatively few characters who are infected with HIV through intravenous drug use is disappointing, as this represents a real risk factor for youth, both in terms of their potential to be exposed to and/or engage in this behavior and/or to be in an intimate relationship with an intravenous drug user. Interestingly, the majority of intravenous drug users presented in these stories are "offstage." They are the mothers of HIV-positive babies, parents who have not been a large part of the protagonist's life, or someone a character used to know. Needle-sharing, the experience of drug use and addiction, and the issues related to the transmission of HIV in injected drug use are not explored in these narratives.

While accidental exposure to HIV-infected blood does represent a real concern, outside of needlesticks in a medical setting and the sharing of needles among drug users, the transmission of HIV through blood or blood products has largely been contained. Nonetheless, blood is the fourth most frequent explanation for transmission of HIV used in these books. The blood supply has been considered clean since 1985; however, books in which blood transfusion is the primary explanation for the transmission of HIV were published as late as 1995. While these stories can be interesting and moving, they do not provide a realistic view of the risks of HIV infection.

As stated above, the risk of vertical transmission is also much lower than it once was; however, there are scenarios in which it is reasonable for readers to expect to find characters who became infected through vertical transmission. For example, in stories set in contexts where prenatal care is limited or unavailable, vertical transmission remains a possibility and is a believable outcome. Likewise, in contexts where medical treatment is available, it is reasonable to expect to see characters who were infected vertically survive to young adulthood. Books that include HIV/AIDS characters who are born in circumstances in which prenatal care is not possible or who have survived to young adulthood both provide realistic scenarios for young adult readers.

WHAT FEARS, IF ANY, DOES THE PROTAGONIST HAVE ABOUT CONTRACTING HIV/AIDS?

This question examines the kind of fears protagonists have about HIV/AIDS both for themselves and others. These fears are also analyzed for whether they are "reasonable" or "unreasonable." Reasonable fears are those that reflect an actual risk of infection and relate to exposure to HIV through sexual contact, blood, or vertical transmission. Reasonable fears can also reflect the social context and may relate to consequences of infection, for example, potential or real violence and social isolation.

Unreasonable fears are concerns the protagonist has that do not reflect a real risk of infection. These fears include being afraid of casual contact with a HIV-infected person and fears of such bodily fluids as saliva and tears, which do not carry the virus. The concern here is whether these texts reflect medical facts and that they do not promote irrational fears or inappropriate social reactions to HIV/AIDS characters.

In this set of novels, it is demonstrated that unreasonable fears dominate the reasons why protagonists fear HIV/AIDS for themselves and others. This is true across all the years of publication considered in this analysis. The emphasis on unreasonable fears coupled with the inattention to the real risks of HIV infection for young adults indicates that this literature is not doing a complete job of providing readers with information about the true risks associated with the transmission of HIV.

While the focus on fears of casual transmission provides content that is easy to refute and also discuss, what young people need to hear and know are the facts associated with behaviors that truly put them at risk. They need explication of what these behaviors are and models of how to handle difficult situations. It is very surprising how little this literature has to say about fears related to intravenous drug use and unprotected sex and how few circumstances where a real risk of transmission is described are accompanied by evidence of reasonable fears.

While the presentation of fears allows, in many cases, for the narrative to refute the need for fear and/or for the reader to follow the protagonist's process of overcoming fear, the usefulness of this aspect of the narratives is limited by the emphasis on reasons for fear that are not reasonable. Likewise, unreasonable fear is not always challenged in these works, and examples of adults responding to HIV/AIDS characters in extreme ways reifies the idea that against all evidence, there may be a reason to have what are considered unreasonable fears.

WHAT IS THE FATE OF HIV/AIDS CHARACTERS?

What happens to people who have HIV/AIDS in these stories illustrates whether HIV/AIDS can be managed or has to result in death. At the beginning of the epidemic, HIV was much feared because it was not well understood and because the infected suffered and died. Today, HIV-positive people who are diagnosed early are living long enough that that they are dealing with the more typical threats to mortality, such as heart disease, instead of dying of AIDS.[3] Improvements in treatment, however, present a different kind of problem in that they have led some to think that infection with HIV is no longer something to worry about. Yet, this is far from true. An attitude of complacency toward HIV infection works against the public good. There is no cure or vaccine for HIV, and treatment is expensive and does not work for everyone. Education, testing, and counseling are still the most important venues for HIV/AIDS prevention.[4]

Is HIV/AIDS Depicted as a Condition That Can Be Controlled?

Content analysis reveals that the majority of the books analyzed include some statement about control and that control messages have been part of these narratives since the first book, *Night Kites*, was published in 1986.[5] The reasons given for why control is possible vary along a continuum of efficacy: There is practical advice aligned with the Centers for Disease Control and Prevention (CDC), messages that are meant to offer hope, and messages that assert control without ever saying what will make control possible.

The most frequent reason codes for control recorded for these narratives are (in order of frequency) the following: treatment is available, maintaining or adopting healthy habits, hope of a future cure, and thinking positively and/or faith. These code categories, except for hope of a future cure, all reflect the advice given by the CDC.[6] These important messages about control, however, represent less than half of the messages presented as reasons why it is possible to live with HIV. One crucial effort toward prevention, education, is given very short shrift in these books. Education as a method of controlling HIV/AIDS is rarely voiced. HIV/AIDS education is modeled in some of these stories as the topic of school assemblies or other efforts to get HIV education to young adults. The effectiveness of these efforts, however, is not assessed for the reader, and is often not demonstrated in the plot.

The balance of the reasons why one can live with HIV offered in these novels tend to be weak messages intended to help

HIV-positive characters cope with their situation. These characters are advised to focus on the fact that they are still healthy, that other people are living with HIV/AIDS, and that they have the benefit of support from friends and family. While these ideas can be reassuring, they do little to advance the idea that it is possible for those infected with HIV to live a normal life.

Another aspect of the idea that it is possible to control HIV has to do with access to treatment, which can be limited by the setting or context within which HIV/AIDS characters find themselves. Books set outside of the developed world depict the HIV epidemic differently than do those set in the developed world. The novels that take place in Africa and Papua New Guinea are set in an atmosphere of suffering and death directly attributed to HIV/AIDS. Such background data as massive graveyards, severely ill people waiting in line for medical care, and overwhelmed hospitals make the point that many people are affected and that HIV infection has deadly consequences.

In novels set in the developed world, if background information about HIV/AIDS is offered, it tends to be supplied in the form of statistics or in the presence of services, for example, AIDS hotlines, that imply the presence of people living with HIV/AIDS. In these books, medical treatment is generally depicted as available, although the quality of life of HIV/AIDS characters is often shown to be onerous, debilitating, and painful. There are instances however, in which the need for health insurance or the dearth of personal funds to support HIV/AIDS treatment is made obvious.

Are HIV/AIDS Characters Depicted as Living with HIV or Dying of AIDS?

The fate of HIV/AIDS characters in the narrative—whether they live or die—is a second measure of the extent to which the idea is present that HIV infection can be managed in the same manner as other chronic diseases. The overall picture of the survivability of HIV/AIDS in these novels is pessimistic. The fate most frequently met by HIV/AIDS characters in these books is that they die or are dying by the end of the book. The next most frequent fate is "unknown." Together these outcomes account for approximately 75 percent of the outcomes for all characters.

Interestingly, HIV/AIDS characters who survive in these stories tend to be young adults, either protagonists or their friends, who have tested positive for HIV infection. Adults are much more likely to die. Lastly, females have better survivability than do males. This finding may reflect the propensity of many of the first books published on this topic to present HIV/AIDS as an adult male problem.

CONCLUSIONS

Returning to the question of what a reader would know about HIV/AIDS if this body of literature were the only source of education a reader had, it is clear that the information provided is incomplete and weak in terms of communicating the risks, issues, and facts that young adults need to keep themselves and people important to them safe. The vague descriptions of who has HIV/AIDS and how they contracted it make the issues HIV/AIDS presents seem remote in the experience of protagonists. When HIV/AIDS happens mainly to people protagonists do not know and little to no information is provided about how these people contracted the illness or what happens to people who have HIV/AIDS, information about HIV remains mysterious. However, the trend to include more HIV/AIDS characters in the young adult age range and more female characters who have HIV/AIDS is a positive one.

Another way this body of literature could be improved as a vehicle for information about HIV/AIDS would be to include more fear messages that relate to reasonable fears and that connect directly to the actual risks young adults are likely to confront. The persistent emphasis on the unreasonable fear of casual contact may have made some sense early in the epidemic, when the scientific facts around HIV/AIDS were seen as more cloudy by the general public, but they do little to advance the current conversation about HIV/AIDS. Narratives are needed that allow young people to see themselves in these stories; provide real information about the risks of HIV infection; model social situations that are difficult to navigate but that put them at risk; and demonstrate socially responsible reactions to people who have

HIV/AIDS. Such additions would make this body of literature a more comprehensive source of information about HIV/AIDS.

Of course, the answer to the question of what these books offer in terms of HIV/AIDS education as a body of literature does not reflect what individual works contribute on their own. To help with the assessment of individual works, part II provides critical annotations of each work analyzed in this content analysis that consider both the accuracy of the HIV/AIDS information it provides as well as an indication of its literary merits.

While there are shortcomings in the presentation of HIV/AIDS provided in this body of literature, overall, very little actual "wrong" information is provided in terms of the medical facts about transmission and the possibility of a cure. While some of the books may contain information that is dated, only three out of the ninety-three books read for this investigation provide clearly wrong information about HIV/AIDS. The first of these, Pike's *The Last Vampire*, presents the idea that HIV/AIDS can be cured with vampire blood.[7] Obviously there is no medical research available to support this claim, and it is reasonable to assume that readers will not take this idea seriously.

On the other hand, McDaniel's *Sixteen and Dying* includes the statement, "Women with AIDS are dying six times faster than men with AIDS. Once a woman is diagnosed with AIDS, her life expectancy is less than thirty weeks."[8] This statement may stem from several news reports during the early 1990s. For example, in 1994, a large study produced by the University of Minnesota School of Public Health demonstrated a greater statistical likelihood for women with AIDS to die as compared to men;[9] however, within this report and in other subsequent work performed at the time it was suggested that the higher rate of fatality for women was the result of women seeking treatment late in their illness and receiving different treatment than men. Access to health care was reported to be one of the big reasons why women's survival rates were lower.[10] Tonisa Clardy summarizes the results of several studies, saying the following:

> "Women die faster" is the most common statement made about women and HIV/AIDS; however, the data clearly shows this is not the case. Women die faster when they have little or no access to testing or when they do not receive the same

> standard treatment and care as men do upon entry into the health care system.[11]

Gayle Roper's *The Mystery of the Poison Pen* also contains content that perpetuates wrong ideas about the transmission of HIV/AIDS.[12] The main HIV/AIDS character in this book is six-month-old Melody, who has been infected through vertical transmission. Melody is in the care of a foster family, and when her HIV-positive status is discovered, it is determined that she can no longer be allowed in the nursery at church with the other babies during services. The Sunday school teacher, a professional nurse, puts a group of twelve-year-olds to work disinfecting the nursery to make it safe. This procedure is not called into question in the narrative. The exact nature of the danger the toys Melody may have touched poses to others is not explained. The CDC clearly states that, "Contact with saliva, tears, or sweat has never been shown to result in transmission of HIV."[13] A further puzzle is why, if Melody poses a real risk to others, is the job of eliminating that risk put in the hands of children?

On the other hand, there are books that do an excellent job of providing information about HIV/AIDS within the context of narratives that are engaging and depict issues young adults face. Among these are *The Mayday Rampage*,[14] *Earthshine*,[15] *My Brother Has AIDS*,[16] *Push*,[17] *Touch of the Clown*,[18] *Playing with Fire*,[19] *The Beat Goes On*,[20] and *Chanda's Secrets*.[21]

Overall, this body of literature does not yet fully address the information needs that young adults have concerning HIV/AIDS. These books only provide HIV education in limited ways. Readers interested in narratives that directly relate to risk factors for young adults will want to choose titles carefully. Stories are still needed that accomplish the following:

- Include HIV/AIDS characters who are people that young adults care about
- Depict risks of transmission that young people are likely to be faced with and model how to handle these situations
- Portray the lives of young people who have or get HIV through vertical transmission, sex, and/or intravenous drug use

- Discuss the need for individuals to know their HIV status through testing, what the practice of safer sex involves, and the importance of HIV education
- Move beyond the issue of fear of casual contact and represent reasonable fears associated with real risks of infection
- Provide realistic views of life with HIV/AIDS
- Depict the challenges of HIV/AIDS for individuals and society
- Model socially responsible behaviors toward people with HIV/AIDS

NOTES

1. Centers for Disease Control and Prevention (CDC), "Universal Precautions for Prevention of Transmission of HIV and Other Bloodborne Infections," 1999. Available at www.cdc.gov/ncidod/dhqp/bp_universal_precautions.html (18 November 2009).
2. AVERT, "Overview of HIV Prevention," September 18, 2009. Available at www.avert.org/prevent-hiv.htm (18 November 2009).
3. Jonathan Weil, "Researchers Project Lifetime Cost and Life Expectancy for Current HIV Care in the United States," November 1, 2006. Available at http://news.med.cornell.edu/wcmc/wcmc_2006/11_01a_06.shtml (18 November 2009).
4. AVERT, "Overview of HIV Prevention."
5. M. E. Kerr, *Night Kites* (New York: HarperTrophy, 1986).
6. Centers for Disease Control and Prevention (CDC), "Living with HIV/AIDS," 2007. Available at www.cdc.gov/hiv/resources/brochures/print/livingwithhiv.htm (9 September 2009).
7. Christopher Pike, *The Last Vampire* (New York: Archway Paperbacks, 1994).
8. Lurlene McDaniel, *Sixteen and Dying* (One Last Wish) (New York: Bantam, 1992), 48–49.
9. Associated Press, "Women with HIV Found to Die Faster Than Men," *New York Times*, Section C, December 28, 1994, late edition.
10. "Studies Show Little Difference in Survival among Men and Women," *AIDS Alert* 8, no. 9 (September 1993): 146–48.
11. Tonisa Clardy, "Women and HIV/AIDS," *PI* (*Project Inform*) *Perspective*, no. 13 (February, 1993): 10–11.
12. Gayle Roper, *The Mystery of the Poison Pen*, East Edge Mysteries, No. 5 (Elgin, IL: Chariot Books/David C. Cook Publishing Co., 1994).

13. Centers for Disease Control and Prevention (CDC), "HIV and Its Transmission," 1999 (last reviewed by the CDC on March 8, 2007). Available at www.cdc.gov/hiv/resources/factsheets/transmission.htm (18 November 2009).

14. Clayton Bess, *The Mayday Rampage* (Sacramento, CA: Lookout Press, 1993).

15. Theresa Nelson, *Earthshine* (New York: Orchard Books, 1994).

16. Deborah Davis, *My Brother Has AIDS* (New York: Jean Karl/ Atheneum, 1994).

17. Sapphire, *Push* (New York: Vintage Contemporaries, 1996).

18. Glen Huser, *Touch of the Clown* (Buffalo, NY: Groundwood, 1999).

19. Henning Mankell, *Playing with Fire*, trans. from Swedish by Anna Paterson (Crows Nest, NSW, Australia: Allen & Unwin, 2002).

20. Adele Minchin, *The Beat Goes On* (New York: Simon & Schuster, 2004).

21. Allan Stratton, *Chanda's Secrets* (New York: Annick Press, 2004).

II

ANNOTATED BIBLIOGRAPHY, 1981–2008

Annotated Bibliography, 1981–2008

Key		
HIV/AIDS Content Scale	*HIV/AIDS Role in Story Scale*	*Literary Quality Scale*
Accurate	Central to plot	Excellent
Accurate but some implausible content	A subplot	Very good
Accurate but dated	Mentioned in passing	Good
Inaccurate		Passable
		Poor

To be included in this bibliography a title had to meet the following criteria:

1. Must have been published between 1981 and 2008.
2. Must be written for young adults ages eleven to nineteen.
3. The main character must be in the eleven to nineteen age range.
4. Must be an English language title.
5. Must include a character who is HIV positive or who has AIDS.
6. Must be a novel.

ARRICK, FRAN. *What You Don't Know Can Kill You.* New York: Bantam Books, 1992. ISBN 0-440-21894-2 (paperback)
HIV/AIDS Content Scale: Accurate
HIV/AIDS Role in Story Scale: Central to plot
Literary Quality Scale: Good

Debra is thirteen years old and feels overshadowed and inconsequential next to her older sister Ellen, who is perfect in every way. Ellen has a boyfriend in college, is getting ready for her prom, and is pretty and popular at school. When a friend of the family is involved in a car accident, Debra arranges a blood drive for him, even though she is too young to donate herself, and it is then that Ellen learns she has been infected with HIV. The girls' parents urge silence on the matter, wary about the potential for the family to be stigmatized. Debra ends up isolating herself out of fear of disobeying her parents, but Ellen has no such compunction. They both end up telling their best friends, who are unequivocally supportive. The suicide of Ellen's boyfriend Jack, however, brings the news out to the larger community, and what was feared regarding stigma to a large extent comes true. Ellen ends up, with the encouragement of her AIDS support group, pursuing an independent life, moving out of her home, and going to community college.

This novel demonstrates clearly that even partners who believe themselves to be monogamous can still be at risk for contracting HIV. Jack believed he was faithful to Ellen, even when he had sex with a prostitute at a fraternity party, because, "It—it was—you know, just sex. That's all, just sex" (p. 56). The novel also demonstrates the importance of social ties in coping with the ramifications of the disease: Jack, who had nothing tying him to the town or to any individuals except Ellen, commits suicide, while Ellen, widely and deeply connected, finds the inner strength to deal with the disease and the stigma after Jack's suicide and the resulting disclosure of her HIV status in a hostile community. [DC]

BABCOCK, JOE. *The Tragedy of Miss Geneva Flowers.* New York: Carroll & Graf Publishers, 2005. [First published by Joe Babcock in 2002.] ISBN 0-7867-1520-0 (paperback)
HIV/AIDS Content Scale: Accurate
HIV/AIDS Role in Story Scale: A subplot
Literary Quality Scale: Very good

Erick Taylor's life has gone steadily downhill since the death of his younger brother. The loss has taken a terrible toll on his family, and Erick is left feeling like he does not fit in his own life. His parents do not understand him, and he is an outcast at school; perhaps God does not even love him. It is not until he meets Chloe, a drag queen, that Erick begins to express his own desire to dress fabulously, have a boyfriend, and escape his dull and oppressive life at school and home; however, dropping out of school, moving in with Chloe, and doing whatever he wants leads to some bad choices and experiences. Erick ends up overcoming a drug addiction and a propensity for negative relationships, learning in time to be self-supporting and to reconcile with his estranged family. Erick's relationship with Chloe is something of a star-crossed love story. Chloe is an important force in saving Erick from himself and helping him through a series of difficulties to find himself and the path that will allow him to create a life that is solidly his own. Erick is committed to sticking by Chloe in his own self-absorbed way.

From the start, Chloe warns Erick that they can only be friends, not lovers. Erick accepts this even though he is deeply in love with Chloe from the moment he first lays eyes on him. The idea of safer sex is not broached in the narrative, which relies mainly on raw experience to make its points. It is eventually revealed that Chloe has AIDS and that is why he refuses to sleep with Erick, although he loves him, too. Chloe lives with an oppressive regimen of medications to keep him alive. Chloe, ever fabulous, gets sicker, recovers, gets sick again, and eventually dies. [MG]

BAER, JUDY. *The Discovery*. Cedar River Daydreams, No. 20. Minneapolis: Bethany House, 1993. ISBN 1-55661-330-X (paperback)

HIV/AIDS Content Scale: Accurate

HIV/AIDS Role in Story Scale: Central to plot

Literary Quality Scale: Poor

In this entry in the Cedar River Daydreams series, sixteen-year-old Lexi and her close friends are shocked to learn that the confident, athletic Nancy, a pediatric nurse, has HIV, but they quickly rally around her. Nancy is the fiancée of quiet Mike, the brother of Lexi's boyfriend Todd. The wedding has been postponed as Mike and Nancy deal with the implications of Nancy's illness. Nancy reveals that she contracted HIV as a promiscuous teen but has since turned her life around by becoming a Christian. She decides to devote herself, while she is still relatively healthy, to educating high school students about the dangers of drugs and premarital sex. Lexi is also worried about her friend Binky, who is being pressured by Harry, her college freshman boyfriend, to have sex with him. Lexi argues that Binky must save herself for marriage and prays on her friends' behalf: "'Oh, Father,' she petitioned aloud. 'Help! My friends need help, *big time*!'" (p. 54). Lexi apparently has some influence (whether with God or Binky is unclear), because Binky finally does the right thing and refuses Harry.

HIV/AIDS is discussed in biology class, a religious youth group forum, and by Nancy herself when she is a guest speaker at Lexi's high school. In each of these opportunities for HIV/AIDS education, some people express fear and/or stigma attitudes and others show support, but the overall message is that Christians must treat people with HIV/AIDS well regardless of how they got the disease and not judge them. The brief inclusion of an "innocent victim," however, a beautiful HIV-positive baby whose mother was infected through intravenous drug use, contradicts this point. [AYG]

BANTLE, LEE F. *Diving for the Moon*. New York: Macmillan Books for Young Readers, 1995. ISBN 0-689-80004-5 (hardcover)
HIV/AIDS Content Scale: Accurate
HIV/AIDS Role in Story Scale: Central to plot
Literary Quality Scale: Good

Sixth grade has just ended, and Bird is looking forward to spending the summer with her best friend, Josh. They have been friends since they were babies, and their families vacation together at a lake. Josh, a hemophiliac, has contracted AIDS through a transfusion. Over the course of the summer, Bird learns to accept that things will change no matter how much she wants them to stay the same. This gentle, rather contemplative novel promotes tolerance in an understated way. For example, there is no fuss over the fact that a gay couple, Bill and Elliot, are also part of the lake community. Another of the book's strong points is that Bird and Josh speak like real kids, in phrases rather than full sentences, since they know each other so well.

Josh develops pneumonia and is hospitalized. Bird thinks about the AIDS pamphlet her father has given her, and processes the information in a way that is accurate and accessible to younger readers. [AYG]

BENNETT, CHERIE, AND GOTTESFELD, JEFF. *University Hospital: Condition Critical*. Book Two. New York: Berkley Jam Books, 1999. ISBN 0-425-17256-2 (paperback)
HIV/AIDS Content Scale: Accurate
HIV/AIDS Role in Story Scale: Mentioned in passing
Literary Quality Scale: Very good

Zoey Appleton and Tristan March are two of the five eighteen-year-old SCRUBS in a prestigious summer program vying for a full scholarship to medical school. They alternately narrate the story. It is clear to everyone but Zoey and Tristan themselves that they are meant for one another. The series seethes with sexual tension around this pair and Summer Everly, the beautiful-but-bitchy southern belle SCRUB who claims Tristan as her own and is intent on winning the scholarship, too. Zoey retaliates by going out with an attractive guy to make Tristan jealous. The clipped, almost telegraphic sentences make the book a page-turner. Disaster strikes when a car drives right into Aesop's, the club where our heroes are partying. Look-alike friends Tisha and Allie are in the car and badly burned. One survives in a coma, and the other dies. Zoey comes up with a clever way to identify the survivor.

This installment introduces Bishop Wilson, the ten-year-old admitted with a fever of unknown origin that turns out to be HIV. Angelic-looking Bishop also suffers from Tourette's syndrome and so is a medical oddity to the doctors and a misery to his roommate, Jerome. All the SCRUBS, in particular Summer, befriend Bishop and the other children in the pediatric ward. [AYG]

BENNETT, CHERIE, AND GOTTESFELD, JEFF. *University Hospital: Crisis Point*. Book Three. New York: Berkley Jam Books, 2000. ISBN 0-425-17338-0 (paperback)
HIV/AIDS Content Scale: Accurate
HIV/AIDS Role in Story Scale: A subplot
Literary Quality Scale: Very good

Zoey Appleton and Tristan March are two of five students selected for SCRUBS, an exclusive mentoring program at Fable Harbor University Hospital (FHUH). The teens shadow doctors throughout the hospital, performing various minor medical and supportive tasks and competing for a scholarship that will be awarded to only one of the participants. This third title in the University Hospital series, told in the alternating voices of Tristan and Zoey, addresses mistaken identities, abusive relationships, love found and lost and found and lost again, and a hostage situation with the threat of a HIV-infected syringe. A deep knowledge of and affection for young adults informs every page, making what could be tedious melodrama into a strangely compelling and only slightly guilty pleasure.

Bishop Wilson is a new pediatric patient at FHUH, brought in with a fever of unknown origin. The origin, it turns out, is HIV infection. His father, who is also HIV positive, infected the boy purposefully with his blood in an effort to get back at the child's mother for being unfaithful. Bishop also has explosive Tourette's syndrome, and it is this (compulsively staring at breasts and shouting obscenities unpredictably) rather than the HIV that alienates him from the other patients and many of the SCRUBS candidates. He is, simply, a child who is hard to like.

The issue of AIDS is actually dealt with in a mature and informative manner. Factual information is skillfully woven into the story line, and the teen SCRUBS respond to Bishop's illness in a matter-of-fact way, taking appropriate precautions but not treating him fearfully. The implausibility of the cause of Bishop's HIV, and the later hostage threat, are balanced by authentic responses on the part of the participants. [DC]

BENNETT, CHERIE, AND GOTTESFELD, JEFF. *University Hospital: Heart Trauma*. Book Four. New York: Berkley Jam Books, 2000. ISBN: 0-425-17404-2 (paperback)

HIV/AIDS Content Scale: Accurate

HIV/AIDS Role in Story Scale: Mentioned in passing

Literary Quality Scale: Very good

In true soap opera fashion, the question of whether Summer, one of the five summer SCRUBS at Fable Harbor University Hospital, was injected in the chest with AIDS-infected blood is answered in a way that only leads to more mystery. In the meantime, romance remains unattainable for all the SCRUBS, who for various reasons are not able to achieve their heart's desires. As it turns out, the syringe did not have AIDS-tainted blood in it after all; furthermore, the assailant, Wilson, the father of pediatric patient Bishop, is not HIV positive either. As the facts accumulate, it becomes less and less clear whether young Bishop really has Tourette's or how he contracted HIV, if his father did not inject him with his own infected blood, as he claimed.

While Dr. Vic assures Tristan that Bishop really is HIV positive, once the hostage situation is diffused, the plot has less to do with Bishop and his interactions with the SCRUBS and more to do with the drama around the question of whether Zoey and Tristan will ever hook up and whether Summer has rigged the competition for the medical school scholarship to ensure that it is hers. The overall sense is that people with HIV/AIDS are to be treated with compassion but also that regardless of the new treatments available, a positive HIV test may still feel like a death sentence. [MG]

BENNETT, CHERIE, AND GOTTESFELD, JEFF. *University Hospital: Prognosis: Heartbreak*. Book Five. New York: Berkley Jam Books, 2002. ISBN: 0-425-18147-2 (paperback)
HIV/AIDS Content Scale: Accurate
HIV/AIDS Role in Story Scale: Mentioned in passing
Literary Quality Scale: Very good

In the latest installment of the University Hospital series, Zoey is stationed on the oncology ward, while Tristan is assigned to a lab where one of the doctors is doing animal research on a vaccine for multiple sclerosis. Here, he befriends Elmo, a chimpanzee animal subject. Summer is apparently innocent of rigging the scholarship competition, although Zoey is still suspicious. Chad hooks up with the love of his life, and Becky decides to leave Fable Harbor University Hospital and the SCRUBS program to be with Rick, who was transferred to another hospital to await a heart–lung transplant. Tristan continues to sleep with Summer and not with Zoey, and things get even more complicated when Tristan's old friend Billie shows up. But when Tristan is mysteriously paralyzed, he is moved to profess his love to Zoey. In the end, they discover that Tristan's paralysis was caused by medicine given to Elmo and passed to Tristan in a scratch. Tristan heals, but we are left wondering who will win the mysterious scholarship award and who the anonymous donor is.

Bishop and his HIV status get only a brief mention in this installment of the series, although with the cause of his HIV in question, he will potentially play a larger role in the next novel, if one is ever published. Safe sex, however, is a recurring theme, especially as Chad enters into a relationship with Eve. The SCRUBS are supportive and hip and have several witty sayings about condoms and safe sex that make it cool to use protection. [DC]

BENNING, ELIZABETH. [Pseudonym for Alida E. Young.] *Losing David*. New York: Harper Paperbacks, 1994. ISBN 0-06-106147-6 (paperback)
HIV/AIDS Content Scale: Accurate
HIV/AIDS Role in Story Scale: Central to plot
Literary Quality Scale: Passable

Fourteen-year-old ice skater Kim Roberts and her parents are forced to leave their hometown when people discover that she has contracted HIV/AIDS from a tainted blood transfusion. Saying good-bye to her best friend Jill and getting acclimated to a new place is hard for Kim, until she gets involved in a romantic friendship with David, a volunteer at Hope House, a counseling center and hospice for young people with chronic illnesses. Kim is surprised to discover that David has leukemia and is also a patient there. David convinces Kim to come out of her shell and enjoy life again. Kim is so used to being shunned herself that she automatically shuns Chelsea, a girl on crutches, who tries to befriend her at school. Kim's deepening relationship with David forces her to look outside of herself to consider others, including Chelsea and Angie, a little girl with leukemia to whom Kim tells stories. Kim loses some of her newfound confidence when first Angie and then David die, seemingly confirming her belief that "friendship just leads to pain" (p. 21), but she has learned how to manage her disease and stand up for herself. The novel ends with Kim's determination to disclose her illness to the school.

Though the fear of being ostracized permeates much of the book, it is gradually replaced by the courage to accept one's circumstances and move on. Many coping mechanisms are described, with particular emphasis on the benefits of developing a positive attitude. Without being overtly didactic, this novel provides plenty of advice on how to live with HIV/AIDS or another chronic disease in a life-affirming way. [AYG]

BESS, CLAYTON. *The Mayday Rampage.* Sacramento, CA: Lookout Press, 1993. ISBN 1-882405-00-5 (hardcover)
HIV/AIDS Content Scale: Accurate
HIV/AIDS Role in Story Scale: Central to plot
Literary Quality Scale: Excellent

After Jess and Molly get in trouble for an article they wrote in their school newspaper, *The Rampage,* they decide to document what led up to the trouble by recording a series of interviews with each other. Angry at the refusal of adults to address sexuality in any way, they had devised a series of articles focused on AIDS. The first article was about a little boy who never got to start kindergarten because of the community's hostility. While the principal was uneasy with it, he allowed the article to go to press; however, when the next issue arrived, featuring prostitutes and explicit anonymous questions and answers regarding HIV infection, the principal pulled the paper and insisted the two keep to safer topics. With the support of their teacher, however, Jess and Molly write one more issue about homosexuality and AIDS and publish it outside the aegis of the school. There are unintended consequences. Violence erupts, Jess is expelled, Molly is suspended, and one of their favorite teachers is outed as homosexual even though Jess attempted to protect his identity.

This is an honest, authentic look at the social ramifications of HIV/AIDS and the impact that forced silence can have on a community, whether it is a school or a city. Facts about HIV are delivered in a hip tone and are naturally woven into the narrative. While Molly's situation in the end feels a bit heavy-handed (she had sex once, before Jess, with a boy who she now knows is homosexual, and contracted HIV as a result), it does effectively convey the message that even good, smart kids can get AIDS. [DC]

BLOCK, FRANCESCA LIA. *I Was a Teenage Fairy.* New York: Joanna Cotler Books/HarperCollins, 1998. ISBN 0-06-027747-5 (hardcover)
HIV/AIDS Content Scale: Accurate
HIV/AIDS Role in Story Scale: Mentioned in passing
Literary Quality Scale: Very good

Teenaged Barbie (named for the doll) Marks has been groomed by her mother, a former beauty queen, to be a model, even though she would much rather be behind the camera than in front of it. Her one source of consolation is tiny Mab, a fairy who has been her friend since childhood. Mab may or may not be real, but, in the tradition of magic realism, she is presented as a real character throughout. When she was eleven, Barbie was abused by a famous photographer, Hamilton Waverly, whose photographs advanced her career. At sixteen, Barbie meets and recognizes Griffin, a boy who had also been victimized by Waverly, and decides that the time has come to expose Waverly as a criminal. The book chronicles Barbie's amorous and other adventures, encouraged by Mab, whose sexual appetite belies her size, in Los Angeles and New York. Barbie gradually becomes as assertive as Mab, who at the end flies off to Ireland with a fairy "biscuit" (hottie) of her own.

The only HIV/AIDS content consists of a homeless man in a Manhattan gutter. Mab picks the pocket of a prosperous-looking businessman and drops the wallet into the homeless man's lap. She notices the man in need and immediately helps him, providing an excellent model in compassion, if not ethics. [AYG]

BROCKTON, QUINN. *Never Tear Us Apart.* A "Queer as Folk" Novel. New York: Pocket Books/Simon & Schuster, 2003. ISBN 0-7434-7613-1 (paperback)

HIV/AIDS Content Scale: Accurate

HIV/AIDS Role in Story Scale: A subplot

Literary Quality Scale: Passable

This book is the backstory to the Showtime drama *Queer as Folk*. It details the first year of college for good friends Michael and Brian, focusing mainly on their sexual experiences, as Michael looks for love and Brian for further conquests. While their day-to-day lives aren't as entwined as they were in high school, they continue to work out issues of jealousy and share their joys and mishaps as well as the details of their love lives.

Throughout the novel, Michael's uncle Vic struggles with AIDS, but while he has bouts in the hospital, each time he is able to recover. The need for safer sex practices is discussed throughout, and Michael has a brief scare when he finds out that a promiscuous young man named Jason, whom he had sex with, is diagnosed as HIV positive. While Brian's sexuality is every bit as predatory as Jason's, he never considers being tested, nor is there any evidence that he feels at risk of infection. Homophobia is a subtheme, but in any risky situation, including the potential for violence, being socially ostracized, or exposure to HIV, Michael and Brian always come away unscathed. [MG]

CARLSON, MELODY. *Notes from a Spinning Planet: Papua New Guinea.* Colorado Springs, CO: WaterBrook Press/Random House, 2007. ISBN 978-1-40000-7145-6 (paperback)
HIV/AIDS Content Scale: Accurate
HIV/AIDS Role in Story Scale: Central to plot
Literary Quality Scale: Poor

Maddie is interested in becoming a journalist, and when her aunt, who is a successful journalist, invites Maddie to join her on a trip to report on Papua New Guinea, Maddie jumps at the chance. But rather than finding a beautiful innocent paradise, the two discover a dark land overtaken by dangerous crime and AIDS. The first place they visit is an AIDS ward, which is understaffed and overcrowded. There they meet Lydia, their primary guide for the duration of their time in Papua New Guinea. Evangelism is a significant thrust in the novel. Maddie reads from the Bible and prays with the patients on the ward at the same time that she pumps them for information that might help her aunt write the article. After they have spent quite a bit of time in Papua New Guinea, Lydia provides them with the angle that Maddie's aunt is looking for in the article. In return, Maddie's aunt offers to put Lydia through medical school, a dream that Lydia has always had but that has been intensified by the fact that she is HIV positive and wants to help others like herself.

When Maddie first encounters patients on the AIDS ward, her fears overcome her common sense. Even though she knows that you cannot catch HIV from being in the same room with somebody, she feels the disease pressing down on her; however, she overcomes her fears to evangelize and make sure these AIDS patients know God and can be forgiven before they meet their maker. While the general facts regarding HIV are accurate, there is a pervasive sense that the reason the problem is so large is because the locals live such hedonistic lives. [DC]

CHASE, BARBARA. *The Silent Killer*. Kingston, Jamaica: Ian Randle Publishers, 2005. [First edition published in 2000. Revised edition published in 2002.] ISBN 976-637-179-2 (paperback)

HIV/AIDS Content Scale: Accurate
HIV/AIDS Role in Story Scale: Central to plot
Literary Quality Scale: Poor

Natasha and her friends struggle with the fact that their bodies are maturing and they do not yet feel emotionally ready to handle the responsibilities associated with being sexually active. Sex is considered sinful, and thoughts of sex and "strange sweet feelings" (p. 14) are tough for these Christian kids to deal with. Natasha and her best friend Jasmine have a pact to tell each other everything if they start dating, but while Natasha is open about her feelings for Shawn, Jasmine is secretive about her relationship with Mike, first denying that she is dating anyone and then denying that they are sexually active. The truth comes out, however, when Natasha discovers that Jasmine has AIDS. Readers should be warned that the manner in which the dialect of Barbados is presented on the page makes the text quite difficult to read.

Although there is some stigma associated with AIDS in this novel, Natasha and her friends have taken it upon themselves to spread the word about prevention and learn how to be compassionate with people who have AIDS. The facts about HIV are accurate, and, in fact, when Natasha is given a mystery to solve (Jasmine's undiagnosed and then undisclosed illness), she connects some disparate pieces of information to arrive at the conclusion that her friend has AIDS. The course of Jasmine's illness is extremely fast. She contracts HIV in her junior year of high school and dies before she is able to start college. This stretches the bounds of believability, when she started out as a very healthy young woman and when the person who infected her remains symptom free. [DC]

CHASE, DAKOTA. *Changing Jamie*. Round Rock, TX: Prizm Books/Torquere Press, 2008. [Copyright 2007.] ISBN 1-60370-351-9 (paperback)

HIV/AIDS Content Scale: Accurate
HIV/AIDS Role in Story Scale: A subplot
Literary Quality Scale: Good

Jamie Waters is a seventeen-year-old boy who wants to come out of the closet but fears the reaction he will get from his homophobic and increasingly aggressive stepfather. Jamie looks to his best friend, Billy, as an out-and-proud role model, even though Billy's scandalous behavior serves to exacerbate the poor relationship he has with his rich, aloof parents. When Jamie is assigned to tutor football star Dylan, his secret crush, he discovers that Dylan has had a crush on him, too. The ensuing relationship is the subject of the novel and the catalyst for the change noted in the title. Jamie's stepfather drunkenly attacks him for being gay, and as a result Jamie's mother sends her husband packing. Jamie otherwise comes out to overwhelmingly sympathetic family and friends. He and Dylan are the most popular couple at the prom.

This novel introduces the phenomenon of "bug chasers" and "gift givers," terms that Jamie looks up on the Internet. Bug chasers are individuals who intentionally try to get infected with HIV on the assumption that they are going to get it anyway. Gift givers are HIV-positive individuals who infect their willing partners through unprotected sex. Jamie is horrified to learn that Billy is a bug chaser. Billy moves in with Robbie, the callous gift giver with whom he has fallen in love, and turns his back on everyone else in his life. When Billy contracts HIV, Robbie discards him. Shaken, Billy admits that he has made a terrible mistake and reconciles with his family. This perhaps overly optimistic ending ensures that Billy will receive proper medical treatment. [AYG]

COHEN, MIRIAM. *Laura Leonora's First Amendment.* New York: Lodestar Books/Dutton, 1990. ISBN 0-525-67317-2 (hardcover)

HIV/AIDS Content Scale: Accurate

HIV/AIDS Role in Story Scale: Central to plot

Literary Quality Scale: Passable

The news is full of the story of an HIV-positive twelve-year-old boy named Tim, who has sued for, and won, the right to attend public school. He will be admitted to one of the local junior highs, but which one is being kept secret. Laura Leonora Fine and her classmates find the idea of AIDS quite frightening, but at the same time, they are not sure exactly how HIV is transmitted or what the real risks are. Laura wonders, "Could my mom and dad get it? At a certain time of the month, for girls, could it find a way to get up in you, because there is blood? Could the whole seventh grade get it if the AIDS boy came to our school?" (p. 26). Unfortunately, in the period leading up to, during, and after the presence of Tim, none of the students presented here receive any information about HIV/AIDS from any of the adults around them. The information gained from her peers about "those skinny balloons" the kids see on the ground leaves Laura confused. "If an AIDS person wants to cry, or do something on you, you mustn't let them. You must use one of those skinny balloons. How? Sort of like a raincoat, probably" (p. 74).

While no misinformation about HIV/AIDS is presented in this novel, it is safe to say that if all a reader knew about HIV came from this novel, they would possess little useable information as a result of reading it. In the end, Laura is able to reach out to Tim by sitting with him at lunch; however, the author, like the adults in this novel, is unable to initiate a much-needed discussion with young people to help them understand the disease and enhance their ability to respond compassionately and without fear to people whose lives are affected by HIV. [MG]

COOPER, MELROSE. *Life Magic*. New York: Henry Holt and Company, 1996. ISBN 0-8050-4114-1 (hardcover)

HIV/AIDS Content Scale: Accurate

HIV/AIDS Role in Story Scale: Central to plot

Literary Quality Scale: Good

Eleven-year-old Crystal feels overshadowed by her talented family, illustrating the difficulty of being a middle sibling with no talent when both of your sisters are stars. To make things worse, it turns out she has a learning disability. When she learns that her beloved Uncle Joe, an artist, is coming from California to live with the family, her joy at the news is marred by her shame, until Uncle Joe tells her he had a hard time in school, too. Crystal's worries about school and talents seem less important with Uncle Joe around, until he tells her he is dying of AIDS. In finding a way through her grief, Crystal also discovers her talent.

While the symptomology of AIDS in the story is accurate enough, it is troubling that no indication of cause is provided for any of the characters, not even deeply veiled hints. No connection is made anywhere between medications, wellness, causes, illness, or death. Uncle Joe purposely skips a dose of his medicine, but there are no consequences, and when he dies, it is from a blow to the head, the result of a seizure. The seizure itself is AIDS related, but the death is random. The overall impression, then, is that AIDS is capricious—it attacks randomly and one is helpless against it. [DC]

DAVIS, DEBORAH. *My Brother Has AIDS*. New York: Jean Karl/Atheneum, 1994. ISBN 0-689-31922-3 (hardcover)
HIV/AIDS Content Scale: Accurate
HIV/AIDS Role in Story Scale: Central to plot
Literary Quality Scale: Very good

Lacy and her brother Jack have a very close relationship, despite the fact that he is twelve years her senior and now living away from home. When the family learns that Jack has AIDS, they struggle with how to manage the situation. Lacy's parents want to keep his HIV status secret, and they are unsure at first whether they want him to move back home, even though he has nowhere else to go. Unfortunately, no one asks Lacy's opinion. She is conflicted but mostly wants Jack to come home. She is unprepared, however, for what the illness does to him, and because the family is so focused on his care, they fail to intervene when Lacy stops swimming, an important activity that had been helping her cope. When Jack dies, Lacy shows her resilience by swimming in the regional meet and helping her team achieve second place.

The AIDS content in this novel is compelling. When we meet Jack, he has already been ill for quite some time, and the impact on Lacy is jarring. We experience each of Jack's symptoms through Lacy's eyes and through the combination of her love and horror. The family is very afraid of stigma, mostly because Lacy's dad "beat up a kid like Jack" (p. 97) when he was a teenager, but when word gets out that Jack has AIDS after a class presentation that Lacy gives, the response is overwhelmingly supportive in spite of a few small instances of stigma attitudes. [DC]

DOCTOROW, CORY. *Little Brother*. New York: Tor Teen, 2008. ISBN-10 0-7653-1985-3 (hardcover)
HIV/AIDS Content Scale: Accurate
HIV/AIDS Role in Story Scale: Mentioned in passing
Literary Quality Scale: Excellent

Extrapolating on recent history, a plausible future unfolds, reflecting the fears of many Americans in the post–9/11 world, in which individual rights are pitted against perceived safety. Marcus is a techie high schooler whose life suddenly becomes centered on the problem of how to bring the government down. There is much to discuss in this text in terms of personal rights and how to preserve them in the face of terrorism. Also of interest is the government's use of surveillance and torture on its own citizens. The use of technology and the positions these young adults assume in protecting traditional American values make this an engaging and informative novel. Readers will also enjoy the many excellent explanations of the math, coding, and logic behind Marcus's understanding of government tactics and his own technological response.

HIV/AIDS is not a theme in this story. Omnipresent surveillance reveals many secrets that would not normally be anyone's business. For example a young person's HIV-positive status is revealed to his parents when he is seen going into a clinic for care. In another discussion, the idea of a super-AIDS virus is used in a math example that explains the "paradox of the false positive" (pp. 128–29) and also explains how infection and transmission occur. This is an excellent book that provides multiple views of important subjects and promotes thinking and discussion. [MG]

DOHERTY, BERLIE. *The Girl Who Saw Lions*. New York: Neal Porter/Roaring Brook Press, 2008. [First published in Great Britain by Andersen Press, Ltd.] ISBN-10 1-59643-377-9 (hardcover)

HIV/AIDS Content Scale: Accurate
HIV/AIDS Role in Story Scale: A subplot
Literary Quality Scale: Good

Abela is a Tanzanian child who has lost both her father and mother to AIDS. Her uncle, who has been living in England illegally, has a plan that involves Abela to gain his legal residency there: He marries his English girlfriend and tries to pass Abela off as their child. His ultimate plan for Abela, however, is to sell her once all the dust has settled. In a parallel story, thirteen-year-old Rosa's mother wants to find a Tanzanian child to adopt. Rosa is upset by this plan, as she is used to having her mother to herself and worries about what this change in their family might mean.

The novel alternates between Abela's and Rosa's lives, inevitably bringing them to each other through a series of unlikely coincidences. While the outcome of this story is fairly predictable, many of the issues that come up in the course of the story—slavery, female circumcision, treatment of the elderly, and government fraud—may be surprising to readers. It is the introduction of these topics that raises the maturity level of this book. Without them, the intended audience would be much younger, as the plot and the telling are both fairly simple.

The majority of the HIV/AIDS content takes place at the beginning of Abela's story and reflects an African landscape reeling from the epidemic, a lack of medicine and health care, and the devastation the disease is bringing to many families. While much is made of the fact that nine-year-old Abela has documentation showing she is AIDS free, the astute reader will wonder what risk of HIV infection she might be facing as a result of being circumcised by the local medicine woman. HIV/AIDS in England is not given much consideration in this story. The main concern is that being HIV positive would make it difficult for Abela to find an adoptive home. [MG]

DOW, UNITY. *Far and Beyon'*. San Francisco: Aunt Lute Books, 2001. [First published by Longman, Botswana Pty., Ltd. in December 2000. This edition published in North Melbourne, Australia, in conjunction with Spinifex Press Pty., Ltd., in 2001.] ISBN 1-879960-64-8 (paperback)

HIV/AIDS Content Scale: Accurate
HIV/AIDS Role in Story Scale: Central to plot
Literary Quality Scale: Very good

Teenagers Mosa and Stan have lost their two older brothers, Pule and Thabo, to AIDS. Such a high death toll among young people is typical in this novel set in contemporary Botswana and written by a human rights activist and judge. The deaths bring Mosa and Stan closer together, and both try to help their mother, Mara, who looks to them for greater involvement in the family's affairs. Mosa struggles with her increasing awareness of how women are devalued in her society, even as schoolgirls, as she and others are set upon by lecherous teachers at their school. She comes up with an ingenious plan to embarrass the teacher who has humiliated her, while directing attention to the issue during a high-profile school visit by the minister of education. Stan is torn between two completely different worlds, the traditional hardworking village life of his impoverished family and his relatively carefree existence with the liberal American teacher with whom he boards.

Dow offers a fascinating insider's look at the AIDS pandemic in Africa. Mara believes AIDS should be treated with traditional African medicine (witch doctors), while her children opt for the Western approach. Mara allows herself to be persuaded by a witch doctor that her close friend Lesedi caused Pule's and Thabo's deaths by bringing evil spirits into Mara's household; thankfully she is reconciled with Lesedi before Cecilia, Lesedi's daughter, dies of AIDS as well. [AYG]

DURANT, PENNY RAIFE. *When Heroes Die.* New York: Atheneum, 1992. ISBN 0-689-31764-6 (hardcover)
HIV/AIDS Content Scale: Accurate
HIV/AIDS Role in Story Scale: Central to plot
Literary Quality Scale: Good

Uncle Rob has AIDS. This is the first in a series of revelations that Gary has to face. It seems that just as Gary needs Rob most—to help with his budding questions about girls and courtship—instead he has to deal with Rob's illness, the disclosure that Rob is gay, and the quickly apparent fact that Rob is dying. Gary cannot believe this is happening to Uncle Rob. After all, Rob is a manly man who drives a cherry red Corvette, was an NCAA basketball player, and anyway, women are always flirting with him. Worse, if Rob is gay, does this mean Gary is, too? Is that why he is so shy around Shanna, the queen of the seventh grade?

While Gary is dealing with all of these questions, Rob's health is rapidly deteriorating. He goes from a healthy athleticism to death in what feels like a few weeks; however, there is time enough for Gary to move from a state of denial to acceptance of both Rob's illness and his sexual orientation, and he is able to connect with Shanna during this time. The HIV/AIDS information provided in this story is minimal, but it does model the use of nonfiction reading as a way to garner information about the disease. While the protagonist is in seventh grade, the overall level of this book is much more suited to younger readers.

As a result, many young adult readers may find it too immature in content to be fully engaging. [MG]

ELIOT, EVE. *Insatiable: The Compelling Story of Four Teens, Food, and Its Power*. Deerfield Beach, FL: Health Communications, 2001. ISBN 1-55874-818-0 (paperback)
HIV/AIDS Content Scale: Accurate
HIV/AIDS Role in Story Scale: Mentioned in passing
Literary Quality Scale: Passable

Each of the sixteen-year-old protagonists in this novel has an eating disorder: Phoebe is obese, Jessica is in the late stages of anorexia, Samantha is in the earlier stages but also self-harms, and Hannah binges and purges. Their stories unfold like case studies as the novel explores each of their support systems and coping mechanisms. Three of the four girls make progress through therapy and/or fortuitous friendships. Jessica, who is hospitalized when her starvation causes a fainting spell in which she cracks her skull, is the only one for whom no adult intervenes, despite the fact that she clearly needs intervention. She continues to decline until anorexia claims her, and it is only her younger brother who seems truly to grieve her loss. Even Phoebe, her best friend, is too absorbed in her own weight problems to spend much time mourning Jessica. The use of Jessica as an object lesson (if you let it, anorexia will kill you) might instead send the unfortunate message that if you're unhappy and lack people in your life who know how to care for you, then the world is probably better off without you.

Jessica's deceased father was a nurse and ostensibly contracted HIV from an accidental needlestick. While it is technically possible to contract the disease in this way, the likelihood has been minimized, given training and universal precautions. There are also rumors that he was homosexual, but Jessica "worked hard at not letting herself visit [the] fear" (p. 35) that he was. Because Jessica's father and his HIV merit only about four sentences in the whole novel, the reader is left with an unsolved mystery and unsatisfying clues. [DC/AYG]

ELLIS, DEBORAH. *The Heaven Shop*. Allston, MA: Fitzhenry & Whiteside, 2004. [Canadian editorial office in Markham, Ontario.] ISBN 1-55041-908-0 (hardcover)

HIV/AIDS Content Scale: Accurate
HIV/AIDS Role in Story Scale: Central to plot
Literary Quality Scale: Very good

Even though thirteen-year-old Binti Phiri stars in *Gogo's Family*, a Malawian radio show about social problems, including HIV/AIDS, she does not make the connection between the disease and her own father's symptoms. The family business (the coffin shop of the title) is booming because so many people are dying of AIDS. Yet, Binti is sheltered from the real impact of the disease until it hits home: Her father dies, and it becomes clear that her mother also died of AIDS six years earlier. As a result, the business is sold, and Binti and her brother and sister pack off to live with relatives who mistreat them. Binti escapes to her grandmother's home, where her Gogo provides food and shelter for many AIDS orphans. The novel follows Binti's progress from a self-absorbed child to a selfless young teen who fully appreciates that the stigma surrounding HIV/AIDS must be overcome and practical help be provided for her community to survive. In this way she becomes a valued member of her own Gogo's family.

Overall this is an absorbing read with well-developed characters. Gogo's young friend, Jeremiah, an HIV-positive peer counselor, is too overtly the mouthpiece of AIDS education. Binti's brother and sister are conveniently paired off with romantic interests; however, the novel offers a nuanced, in-depth look at the AIDS pandemic, including the roles of prostitution and imprisonment. Canadian writer and social activist Ellis visited Malawi and Zambia for her research. Illustrator Janet Wilson's cover and frontispiece are inviting and culturally appropriate. The book concludes with an author's note about AIDS and Sub-Saharan Africa and a brief interview with Ellis. [AYG]

FIELD, BARBARA. *The Deeper, the Bluer*. Lincoln, NE: iUniverse .com, 2000. ISBN 0-595-13378-9 (paperback)
HIV/AIDS Content Scale: Accurate
HIV/AIDS Role in Story Scale: A subplot
Literary Quality Scale: Passable

Five single female friends in San Diego, California, rely on each other as they navigate mainly troubled relationships with men over the course of roughly a year. Several social issues, including bisexuality, domestic violence, and HIV/AIDS are integral to the story. The young adult protagonist, Claire, has lost her father to AIDS and copes with the impending loss of her mother, who is HIV positive, by attempting to get pregnant by the son of one of her mother's friends. Her boyfriend's mother, Molly, has left an abusive relationship. Claire babysits for Dorie, an untamed, selfish mother of two, and Renata, a successful lawyer who has just kicked her husband out. Summertime brings them all together around the community swimming pool, and Claire, unsure of whether she is pregnant and afraid to find out, examines the different manifestations of single motherhood, trying to determine if she wants to join their ranks. The feminization of poverty, the disadvantages women face in seeking help through the legal system, and the support of female friendship are explored in the narrative, which offers little in terms of the kind of deep connection Claire seeks in her relationship with others.

Drug use and bisexuality are the causes of HIV infection in this story, but Claire does not ponder any risk associated with engaging in unprotected sex in the hope of becoming pregnant. Claire's mother, Virginia, was infected by her husband, but the possibility of HIV infection is not discussed among the women. Virginia's AIDS is just one problem in a novel rife with problems that should be deep and emotional but end up shallow and lacking affective impact. Everyone but Virginia treats her HIV status in a completely matter-of-fact manner, as though AIDS were as catastrophic as a hangnail. Facts about HIV/AIDS treatments and the course of the disease are both realistic and fatalistic, and although Claire's mother is alive at the end of the story, it is also clear that she is dying. As with other social issues embedded in this narrative, the cost of medical care and the need for adequate health insurance are touched on but not fully explored. [DC/MG]

FIRST BORN. [Pseudonym for Brian Williams.] *Delivered from Evil.* Bloomington, IN: Trafford Publishing, 2006. ISBN 1-4120-8048-7 (paperback)

HIV/AIDS Content Scale: Accurate

HIV/AIDS Role in Story Scale: Mentioned in passing

Literary Quality Scale: Poor

Set in Tallahassee, Florida, this novel written in interconnected short stories chronicles how twelve young people, mostly African Americans, become disciples of the born-again Reverend

James Dawkins. Each, including Dawkins, has reached a turning point after a terrible experience due to a lifestyle of hedonism and/or criminal activity.

The single instance of HIV/AIDS comes up in the disciple Darius's story. Darius is promiscuous; he has been intimate with ninety-seven women in five years. In a dream, one of his current girlfriends, Dedra, appears at his funeral and tearfully tells him that she did not reveal her HIV-positive status when they met. Because Darius has dreams that come true, it is implied that in several months he will be dead; however, from the epilogue it is clear that he survives. The dream episode is the turning point that saves him. Contracting HIV/AIDS, then, is presented as one of a number of horrific possible consequences of an ungodly life. [AYG]

FLINN, ALEX. *Fade to Black*. New York: HarperTempest, 2005. ISBN 0-06-056839-9 (hardcover)
HIV/AIDS Content Scale: Accurate
HIV/AIDS Role in Story Scale: Central to plot
Literary Quality Scale: Excellent

Early one morning, seventeen-year-old Alejandro (Alex) Crusan, widely know to be HIV positive, is attacked in his car by a baseball bat–wielding young man who smashes the windshield. Alex and his family are Cubans who have recently moved to the small-town, less-than-welcoming fictional community of Pinedale, Florida, from the more cosmopolitan Miami. Daria, a Down Syndrome student who has a crush on Alex, identifies their bigoted classmate, Clinton Cole, as the culprit. Clinton denies that he did it, although he has harassed Alex and his family before. The story is told in the voices of these three characters. Alex is believable as a young man struggling to carry on his life in an ordinary way under extraordinary circumstances. Daria's thoughts are expressed in a very spare, poetic text. The author, an attorney who has worked on cases involving young people and various types of abuse, is particularly adept at getting inside the head of delinquent young men in her novels. Not surprisingly, Clinton dominates this book, which is more an anatomy of a bully than a whodunit, since we learn fairly early on that Clinton is not the attacker—this time.

HIV/AIDS is presented through the superstitions spouted by Clinton and his friends and matter-of-fact, accurate information from Alex and others. The text focuses on how people treat Alex as a person, not on how he got infected; the latter is the real mystery of the story. We do not discover until the end that, contrary to his mother's public insistence that he contracted the disease through a blood transfusion (which no one believes anyway), he actually got it through unprotected heterosexual sex. This is an uncompromising, absorbing read. [AYG]

FOX, PAULA. *The Eagle Kite.* New York: Orchard Books, 1995. ISBN 0-531-06892-7 (hardcover)
HIV/AIDS Content Scale: Accurate
HIV/AIDS Role in Story Scale: Central to plot
Literary Quality Scale: Passable

Liam Cormac is thirteen when he learns that his father is infected with HIV as the result of a homosexual relationship. Liam is initially told that his father was infected as a result of a blood transfusion following appendicitis, but he recognizes the lie, and it forces him to rethink his family dynamics at the same time that he is trying to cope with his father's HIV. Liam must come to terms not only with his father's illness but also with shame related to his father's homosexuality. The antigay sentiment is pervasive and only incompletely resolved here—conservative parents may be comfortable with it, but questioning youth will find a hostile environment.

The facts about HIV/AIDS are accurately presented through the medium of health classes, Liam's own research after learning of his father's illness, and Liam's observations of his progressively ill father. Other potential causes are mentioned (in fact, Liam would prefer that his father were infected via intravenous drug use rather than homosexual sex), but as a result of the antigay sentiment in the book, it represents and reinforces the stereotype of HIV being a gay man's disease. [DC]

GLEITZMAN, MORRIS. *Two Weeks with the Queen.* New York: Putnam, 1991. [First published in Australia by Penguin Books Australia, Ltd. in 1989.] ISBN 0-141-31455-9 (paperback)
HIV/AIDS Content Scale: Accurate
HIV/AIDS Role in Story Scale: A subplot
Literary Quality Scale: Excellent

Colin's feelings are hurt when his younger brother Luke gets a toy for Christmas and he gets a pair of new shoes instead of the microscope he was hoping for; however, when Luke is diagnosed with leukemia, Colin agrees to go visit family in England so that he can carry out his secret plan to enlist the help of the Queen in locating "the best doctor in the world" (p. 83) to save his brother. In Colin's dogged pursuit of a way to save Luke he meets Ted Caldicot, whose lover, Griff, is dying of AIDS. Through the remarkable friendship that develops between Colin and Ted, Colin begins to understand what his brother Luke really needs from him and undertakes another secret plan.

Told with both extraordinary humor and tenderness, the parallel plots of Luke's leukemia and Griff's AIDS, both incurable, demonstrate the human dimension of illness. Information about HIV/AIDS is given in a matter-of-fact manner. Colin is not afraid to meet and visit with Griff in the hospital and, while homophobia is demonstrated in the story, Colin accepts the idea that two men can be in love without feeling threatened by it. While overall Colin is surrounded by ineffectual adults who provide neither information nor solace, his trip to England to meet the "queen," who can help, is not to be missed. [MG]

GONZALES, S. BRYAN. *Under the Big Sky*. Bloomington, IN: AuthorHouse, 2006. ISBN-10 1-425-96524-5 (paperback)
HIV/AIDS Content Scale: Accurate
HIV/AIDS Role in Story Scale: Mentioned in passing
Literary Quality Scale: Passable

Cash is a rodeo hero and Travis a football star. They come from different worlds but go to the same high school, and their mutual attraction is undeniable. Their relationship is also quite stormy, however, rife with secrecy and jealousy. Lee, a rodeo man with a bad reputation but a great body, tempts Cash. And Travis must deal with his mother throwing his ex-boyfriend Jason at him, although that relationship has been over for some time. Short paragraphs and melodramatic language would ordinarily indicate a fast-paced story, but in this case the reader is taken in brief syncopated hops through every moment, every random thought, every dropped fork, of every single day. What might otherwise be an engaging story ends up being twice as long as necessary and thus hardly engaging.

When Travis's mother funds a visit from Travis's ex-boyfriend, Jason, in an attempt to get her son's mind off of Cash, Travis learns not only that Jason was cheating on him when they were together but also that Jason is now HIV positive. Since there is no way to know when Jason contracted the disease, Travis must be tested. While Cash is initially afraid for Travis and himself, there is no discussion of the two practicing safer sex once they learn that Travis has dodged that particular bullet. In addition, Cash cheats on Travis with Lee, and there is no mention of protection at any point. [DC]

GOODMAN, ALISON. *Singing the Dogstar Blues*. New York: Viking, 2002. [First published by Voyager, an imprint of HarperCollins Publishers Australia, in 1998.] ISBN 0-670-03610-2 (hardcover)

HIV/AIDS Content Scale: Accurate but some implausible content
HIV/AIDS Role in Story Scale: Mentioned in passing
Literary Quality Scale: Excellent

In the future, the secrets of time travel have been unlocked, but only a select few are trained in its mysteries and dangers. Joss is one of these elites, a new student at the Center for Neo-Historical Studies. Mav, Joss's partner and dormmate, is the first alien ever to be admitted to the school, and some are not pleased about the alien's presence. Complicating the situation is the fact that the Chorians are a twinned species, and Mav lost his twin in an accident. When Mav becomes ill as a result of pining for his lost twin, Joss decides that the only way to save him, never mind the rules, is to go back in time and alter the events that led to Mav's loss. What the two discover changes them forever. The plotting in this novel is tight and compelling, and every detail is used to its fullest capacity. In addition, the developing friendship between Joss and Mav is filled with delightful moments, some laugh-out-loud funny and some tender and sweet.

HIV content in this novel is minimal. There is a museum that Joss ducks into after she has escaped school for the day. This museum holds what remains of the AIDS quilt, much of which was destroyed in a fire after gay marriage was legalized many years prior. Interestingly, a new strain of HIV has emerged, related to elective brain implants intended to increase intelligence. Visitors to the museum are rare, and no additions to the quilt have been made in more than fifty years, although people still contract HIV. The museum director laments, "Maybe people have just forgotten" (p. 132). [DC]

HANSEN, JOYCE. *One True Friend.* New York: Clarion, 2001. ISBN 0-395-84983-7 (hardcover)

HIV/AIDS Content Scale: Accurate
HIV/AIDS Role in Story Scale: A subplot
Literary Quality Scale: Good

Amir's primary goal in life is to reunite his siblings after they get separated following the death of their parents. He moves from place to place, stopping for a while in the Bronx and becoming good friends with Doris, and ending up in the home of the foster parents who have adopted his youngest brother. While he is living there, he corresponds regularly with Doris, who supports him both in his search for his remaining lost siblings and in his struggle to belong in the foster family that has taken him in. The story focuses primarily on his experience, although Doris and the town in which Amir spent some time earlier do feature prominently. Her letters to him are full of gossip about people he knew, interspersed between copious amounts of encouragement and advice.

Amir's parents died of AIDS caused by intravenous drug use. Amir has quite a bit of shame surrounding the circumstances of their deaths, but when he reveals to Doris that they died of AIDS and not in a car accident, as he had originally told her, she is supportive and accepting. The facts surrounding HIV are accurate, such as they are, but there is very little content here. He admits that his parents died of AIDS and that they were junkies. Doris says, "Okay," and they move on to the next thing. This novel can perhaps be recommended more as a model for compassionate response than as a text from which to glean much pertinent information regarding HIV and AIDS. [DC]

HARLEY, REX. *Now That I've Found You.* Llandysul, Ceredigion, Wales: Pont Books/Gomer Press, 2003. ISBN 1-85902-107-7 (paperback)

HIV/AIDS Content Scale: Accurate
HIV/AIDS Role in Story Scale: A subplot
Literary Quality Scale: Excellent

In this delightfully British novel, the narrator, a college-aged boy (the American equivalent would be high school) meets a mysterious and compelling girl who claims to be visiting from the past. She will not even tell him her name, and although we eventually learn she is Rhiannon, we never do learn the narrator's name—a brilliant and satisfying subtlety. The narrator is raised by his father after his mother is killed in a train accident, but although the narrator is hungry to know more about his mother, it is a subject his father will not address, ostensibly out of grief. So, the mystery of his mother is braided into the mystery of the new girl in his life. In a series of epiphanies, he discovers that Rhiannon is HIV positive, the result of a rape when she was younger; and that his mother and father never married—his father's silence was based on shame and a wish not to taint the narrator's sense of self, rather than solely on grief, as the narrator had believed. While these situations sound melodramatic, they are actually treated with a deft hand, providing a deeply satisfying reading experience.

Rhiannon's HIV status and the rape that led to her contracting HIV is not revealed until the novel is nearly at an end, yet it is treated fully and with profound insight into the experience both of those who have HIV and those who love them. The fears are raw and visceral, the hope is heartbreaking, and the lifestyle adjustments, both small and large, are honest and poignant. [DC]

HERMES, PATRICIA. *Be Still My Heart*. New York: G. P. Putnam's Sons, 1989. ISBN 0-671-70645-4 (paperback)
HIV/AIDS Content Scale: Accurate
HIV/AIDS Role in Story Scale: A subplot
Literary Quality Scale: Passable

High school sophomore Allie Dalton agrees to let her best friend Leslie make Allie over into a thinner, sexier person who will be attractive to someone other than nerdy Ronald Hamburger. Allie has privately set her sights on dishy David, who works with her on the school newspaper. Leslie, however, tries to fix her up with David's cousin, Mark, the handsome new boy in town, because Leslie is taken with David herself. Allie does not want to interfere with what she sees as the romance between David and Leslie. Predictably, we learn that David is in fact more interested in Allie, and Leslie ends up with Mark, but in the midst of this game of romantic musical chairs, something serious is happening at school. Allie's favorite teacher, Ms. Adams, is in danger of losing her job because her husband has been diagnosed with HIV/AIDS, which he contracted through a blood transfusion some years earlier. The immediate crisis is averted because Ms. Adams consults a lawyer and realizes that the school board has no grounds to dismiss her. It is up to Allie, however, to encourage an atmosphere of acceptance by writing an article about HIV/AIDS and discrimination for the school paper and organizing an assembly for students to meet Mr. Adams and see that he is just a regular guy.

Information about HIV/AIDS is presented accurately as Allie does her research and has discussions with knowledgeable adults; however, in spite of all the AIDS education courses Allie has had at school, she is initially fearful about transmission through casual contact—not with the person with HIV/AIDS but with his spouse. This response is not really prompted by anything and is jarring to the reader. On the other hand, even though she is immature for her age, Allie's fears about future sexual encounters are realistic. Although the threats in this book tend to just melt away—apparently the article and the assembly solve the problem—the depiction of Ms. Adams's vandalized car and the conversation of ignorant kids at school who assume that Mr. Adams must be a "queer" demonstrate that stigma is alive and well. [AYG]

HERNÁNDEZ, IRENE BELTRÁN. *Woman Soldier/La Soldadera*. Waco, TX: Blue Rose Books, 1998. ISBN 0-9676833-0-0 (paperback)

HIV/AIDS Content Scale: Accurate

HIV/AIDS Role in Story Scale: A subplot

Literary Quality Scale: Poor

Nico Lorenzo's junior year at Pinkerton High School is full of surprises for her and for the reader. Nico, a loner, is called the Woman Soldier in the barrio where she lives. Her sole companion is a ghost called Angelica, also a fighter, whom only she can see. Nico joins the Reserve Officers' Training Corps (ROTC) for the uniform but soon discovers she has a talent for military drills. Even better, if she can improve her grades, she will be eligible for a scholarship to West Point. While she finds her ROTC gringo tutor, Ryan, very attractive, it is the even more handsome Reyno, a former enemy and current gang leader, with whom she falls in love. Nico demands that Reyno choose between her and the gang. The characters' motivations are often unconvincing and even bizarre. Why would Nico, a self-described rebel, suddenly opt for military discipline? Reyno broke Nico's nose in a fight when she was twelve and apparently has not talked to her since, but now, five years later, he declares his long-standing love. Ms. Rendon, the intelligent and caring librarian, says that Reyno could not possibly be in danger from his gang because he is handsome. Such oddities make this novel read like an early draft.

Both of Nico's parents died of AIDS when she was about five. Her father was in prison, where he contracted the disease and unknowingly passed it on to his wife during a conjugal visit. After her mother's death, Nico was raised by her grandparents. Even though it killed her mother and father, Nico only momentarily wonders if she could get AIDS from Reyno, should they have sex. In this book, AIDS is relegated to the past. [AYG]

HOBBS, VALERIE. *Get It While It's Hot. Or Not.* New York: Richard Jackson/Orchard, 1996. ISBN 0-531-09540-1 (hardcover)
HIV/AIDS Content Scale: Accurate
HIV/AIDS Role in Story Scale: A subplot
Literary Quality Scale: Good

Megan Lane and her three friends, Kit, Mia, and Elaine, all high school juniors, are self-proclaimed "friends till the end" (p. 1). Megan's mother, a high-powered pediatric nurse, has always discouraged Megan's friendship with Kit, a girl who seems to invite disaster. Kit becomes pregnant, is diagnosed with toxemia, and must stay in bed. The friends rally round Kit to care for her, since her alcoholic mother is seldom home and is quite ineffective when she is. Megan must help out secretly because of her mother's disapproval. Megan has been writing an exposé about teen sex for her high school newspaper, and Kit's situation only convinces her of the importance of making sure students have accurate information. When the principal refuses to run the story, Megan finds herself once again doing something in secret, surreptitiously publishing the article by distributing photocopies.

Monk, the school football star and, after a single tryst, the father of Kit's baby, has contracted HIV/AIDS through sharing a needle to shoot up steroids. Although Kit and the baby are not infected, the text is ambiguous about the health of Tiffany, Monk's steady girlfriend. Megan's article dispels myths about

HIV/AIDS. Although this novel does not show the course of the disease (Monk is still healthy at the end), it makes a strong case for education as a deterrent. [AYG]

HOFFMAN, ALICE. *At Risk*. New York: Putnam, 1988. ISBN 0-399-13367-4 (hardcover)
HIV/AIDS Content Scale: Accurate
HIV/AIDS Role in Story Scale: Central to plot
Literary Quality Scale: Good

Amanda is a talented gymnast in a family that is falling apart at the seams. When she is diagnosed with HIV, this serves to further isolate the family members from each other and the entire family from the general community. Amanda and her parents find solace in relationships outside the home, but Charlie, Amanda's younger brother, is left completely isolated. His best friend Sevrin is removed from school to "protect" him from Amanda's illness, and he is forbidden to spend time with Charlie, although the two have been best friends since they were born. The principal of the school proves to be a staunch and levelheaded ally, and Amanda is allowed to remain in school despite community protest—as a result, however, many parents pull their children out of the school and stigma continues. The tone of detachment in this novel sometimes belabors the point of the family's lack of solid ties with each other and the community. In the end, however, when Sevrin tries to reconnect with Charlie, the reader is provided with enough tentative hope to redeem, at least partially, the prior disconnection and despair.

While the facts regarding AIDS are accurate in this novel, the progression of the disease is unrealistically quick. Amanda is diagnosed a week before school starts in early September and is dead before Thanksgiving of that same year. This, in an otherwise extremely healthy young girl, a champion gymnast. [DC]

HOOD, ROB N. *Beyond the Wind*. Binghamton, NY: Southern Tier Editions/Harrington Park Press/Haworth Press, 2004. ISBN 1-56023-482-2 (paperback)
HIV/AIDS Content Scale: Accurate
HIV/AIDS Role in Story Scale: Central to plot
Literary Quality Scale: Poor

Christopher's best friend and lover, Kyle, is outed at school and attacked by fellow students—a predictable outcome in conservative Lincoln, Nebraska. Kyle is forced by his parents into "straightening" therapy. He despairs and runs away to the big city, Omaha, with the intention of becoming a prostitute. When Chris and his friends Jen and Bryce make a road trip to Omaha to retrieve Kyle, they become embroiled in a political intrigue and two murders somehow connected with distinguished senator and AIDS activist Martin Ash. Not surprisingly, when Kyle returns from Omaha he tests positive for HIV. Throughout the story Chris fears that God cannot love him because he is gay, but he is eventually comforted by theological conversations with the doctor who tests him for HIV/AIDS. Although the author's attempt to support GLBT (gay lesbian bisexual transgender) youth in an intolerant world is laudable, it does not make for good literature.

Religious response to HIV/AIDS is a major theme. Several unpleasant characters in this novel believe that HIV/AIDS is visited upon gays as a punishment from God. The author, a youth worker, uses a heavy hand to convince the reader that this is not the case. Chris and his friends sit through a long debate between Ash and a senator from the Christian right, Landan, about a proposal to stop an AIDS prevention program from being incorporated into the Omaha public school system. Ash draws on religion to eloquently defend the program in the face of Landan's religious intolerance. Although an obvious risk to Chris, the promiscuous and selfish Kyle is hurt that Chris refuses to have sex with him. Another character with HIV/AIDS, Nick, a gay security guard who works for Ash, is depicted as a decorated war veteran and a noble soul who fell afoul of the military when he fought in vain to get financial and medical benefits for his partner, who subsequently died of AIDS. [AYG]

HUMPHREYS, MARTHA. *Until Whatever*. New York: Clarion Books, 1991. ISBN 0-395-58022-6 (hardcover)
HIV/AIDS Content Scale: Accurate
HIV/AIDS Role in Story Scale: Central to plot
Literary Quality Scale: Good

Issues of HIV/AIDS and issues of class are intermingled in this novel featuring Connie Tibbs, an HIV-positive high school junior who is from the wrong side of the tracks. Connie was a good friend to her classmate (and the book's protagonist), Karen Thompson, some years earlier when Karen needed a friend. Karen's mother objected to the friendship at the time because she did not approve of Connie's lower-class family. Now that Connie is ill, Karen wants to renew the friendship; however, that means alienating her best friend, Rae, and her boyfriend, Todd. Karen's dilemma is further complicated by the fact that Connie once saved Karen's life. Connie has made it clear that Karen should not feel obligated to her, but their shared history is a constant undercurrent. Karen decides to stick by Connie, doing the right thing rather than the popular thing, and she goes so far as to abandon her cheerleader duties and show up dateless at homecoming. She gradually becomes stronger in her resolve in spite of having become a social pariah. The climax of the book is a shocking episode in which Connie faints, the school nurse refuses to help, and Karen somehow manages to get Connie to the hospital.

Although the plot is quite conventional, the HIV/AIDS content gets a more novel treatment. Karen and Connie play a little game in which they try to come up with "one good thing about AIDS" (p. 91). For example, if you have AIDS, you don't have to diet. This dark humor serves as a coping mechanism as the girls are increasingly isolated at school. Another nuanced way in which the author imparts HIV/AIDS information is through Karen's front-page article for the school newspaper. Although such articles are not unusual devices, Karen's approach is far more thoughtful than most. She ties the students' need to stigmatize Connie to their desire to be safe. If Connie were promiscuous and brought the disease upon herself, then the students could blame her and not worry about their own actions; however, as Karen points out, Connie is not promiscuous, so indeed everyone is at risk. [AYG]

HUNT, ANGELA ELWELL. *A Dream to Cherish*. Cassie Perkins Series, No. 4. Lincoln, NE: Authors Guild Backinprint.com Edition/iUniverse.com, 1992. [First published by Tyndale House Publishers, Inc.] ISBN 0-595-08995-X (paperback)

HIV/AIDS Content Scale: Accurate

HIV/AIDS Role in Story Scale: Central to plot

Literary Quality Scale: Passable

Cassie Perkins changes schools for a year after her parents' divorce. As the novel begins, Cassie has returned to the school that should have been hers from the beginning to find that her friends have changed in her absence. Arien, a girl who has just moved into the area, is instantly popular because she's beautiful and exotic. She inexplicably befriends Cassie, now an outsider, and the two become inseparable despite their difference in age and life experience. When Cassie discovers that Arien has HIV as the result of "when she was younger, when [she] was doing drugs" (p. 146), Cassie is conflicted between wanting to be a good friend to Arien, who needs her, and wanting to get back in good graces with her old group of friends, who are nasty. In the end, she conquers her fears and stays by Arien's side.

The course of the disease is fairly rapid, taking Arien from a hale, healthy roller skating champion to dead in less than a year. In addition, the stigma, presented as a matter of course, is over the top for the time in which it takes place. Cassie's own mother completely rejects her simply for befriending someone with AIDS; she also refuses to listen to reason, being more concerned, erroneously, about the health of her pregnancy than about Cassie's well-being. And at a time when universal precautions were solidly in place, the nurse at Arien's bedside as she is dying wears a "helmet . . . connected to a backpack . . . long-sleeved suit, gloves, long pants, and even had plastic covers on her shoes" (p. 185) and is still reluctant to touch Arien. The novel does not make it completely clear that Cassie's mother and the nurse are acting crazy. There are no consequences for this behavior, and no one really fights it. In the end, this is a novel that engenders fear and hostility toward HIV and its victims and not toward the people who would victimize them. [DC]

HUSER, GLEN. *Touch of the Clown*. Buffalo, NY: Groundwood, 1999. [Canadian editorial office in Toronto.] ISBN 0-88899-343-9 (hardcover)

HIV/AIDS Content Scale: Accurate

HIV/AIDS Role in Story Scale: Central to plot

Literary Quality Scale: Excellent

The improbably named Barbara Stanwyck Kobleimer (thirteen) and her little sister, Olivia de Havilland (seven), called Livvy, find an unexpected friend and protector in Cosmo, the HIV-positive young man who invites them to join his clown workshop. Barbara has been looking after her severely dysfunctional family since the death of her mother and, poignantly, does not even realize how negligent her movie-mad, alcoholic father and grandmother have been. In particular, Barbara has been in charge of Livvy, whose kidney problems result in frequent "accidents." Although this is a grim scenario, it is leavened by the book's many comic touches and moments of genuine friendship. The book ends on a note of guarded optimism: Cosmo dies, but Barbara has absorbed the life lessons he taught her and feels better able to deal with a first boyfriend, new school, and second chance at being young.

This first novel by a Canadian writer, who went on to win the Governor-General's Award for *Stitches*, accurately shows how a responsible young man in an urban environment (likely Edmonton, Alberta) lives with HIV/AIDS. Cosmo discusses his condition in a matter-of-fact manner, and Barbara has no hesitation about being friends with him. As suggested by the cover image of the girls watching Cosmo juggle, the content is particularly suited to younger teens. [AYG]

JOHNSON, SCOTT. *Overnight Sensation.* New York: Atheneum, 1994. ISBN 0-689-31831-6 (hardcover)
HIV/AIDS Content Scale: Accurate
HIV/AIDS Role in Story Scale: Mentioned in passing
Literary Quality Scale: Good

Spending the summer with her cousin changes Kerry's life. Dropping a few pounds and adopting a new hairdo are enough to change her destiny back at home. The popular kids are suddenly interested in her, and it is a heady feeling, so heady that she finds herself unable to counter their anti-Semitic comments or keep herself from participating when they sneak into empty houses to party. Kerry does not stop them when they plan their next rendezvous at her lifelong friend's house while the family is out of town. She does not stop them when they cover the garage wall with "things about Jews" (p. 55) and set the place on fire. Kerry continues to protect them and herself even as they plan their next party in the basement of a house belonging to an old woman who is another important figure in her life. The main theme of this work is the price of compliance traded for superficial ends.

HIV/AIDS is not much of an issue for the characters in this novel. It comes to the fore when Kerry helps to set up an assembly about AIDS. While she does a bad job of making the arrangements, the obviously ill HIV-positive speaker does a good job of making his points to the audience. More directly interesting in terms of HIV/AIDS content in this story, however, is Kerry's inability, try as she may, to get any of her love interests to wear a condom. The question of how to navigate this territory is one readers will be interested in and hopefully will be better able to navigate than Kerry, who always eventually gives in to unprotected sex against her better judgment. [MG]

KAYE, MARILYN. *Real Heroes.* New York: Harcourt Brace Jovanovich, 1993. ISBN 0-15-200563-3 (hardcover)
HIV/AIDS Content Scale: Accurate
HIV/AIDS Role in Story Scale: Central to plot
Literary Quality Scale: Good

Kevin is an average kid caught in the crossfire of his parents' divorce. His mother has left the family. Kevin idealizes his policeman father and thus feels great pressure to agree with his point of view; however, to the reader, Kevin's father appears immature and hotheaded. The need to please his father jeopardizes his relationship with his mother and also with a favorite teacher, Mr. Logan, who is the only adult Kevin feels he can freely talk to. When it is revealed that Mr. Logan is gay and HIV positive, Kevin's father becomes an active member of the parent group determined to drive Mr. Logan away. Even though Kevin does not like the stance his father has taken, he feels that he has to go along with it—but he secretly roots for Mr. Logan's cause.

The plot structure of this novel is one that is familiar in young adult novels that discuss HIV/AIDS. A beloved teacher is HIV positive, and a battle ensues in which stigma around homophobia and HIV/AIDS rages. All of the drama, however, involves adults, perhaps giving the message that HIV/AIDS itself is not a risk or issue for young people, outside of the need to develop tolerance. While the information about HIV/AIDS in this book is accurate as far as it goes, the final chapter, "Further Information about AIDS and HIV," which points readers to various information sources, is understandably dated. [MG]

KERR, M. E. *Night Kites*. New York: HarperTrophy, 1986. ISBN 0-06-447035-0 (paperback)

HIV/AIDS Content Scale: Accurate

HIV/AIDS Role in Story Scale: Central to plot

Literary Quality Scale: Excellent

This is the first young adult novel published that contains an HIV-positive character. It is the story of Erick who falls in love for the first time—with his best friend's girl—while at the same time learning that his idealized older brother, Pete, is gay and has contracted HIV. The family does not take the news about Pete very well, and the text provides a realistic depiction of a family under stress as they cope with both loss and stigma. In fact, coping with Pete's illness rocks the family to the core as they work to keep their private life private and yet still suffer various kinds of social disgrace. Erick is increasingly isolated as the story progresses. He loses his best friend and girlfriend when he takes up with a girl named Nikki. Then he loses Nikki when she finds out about his brother.

While the HIV/AIDS content in this story is accurate, the issues it does not confront head on but that hover in the background are interesting and worthy of discussion. Erick and Nikki never discuss safe sex, even though she has clearly had other partners; furthermore, one of her previous beaus is in jail for drug dealing. Why is it that Erick, whose brother has AIDS and who has read all the pamphlets, does not feel any personal risk of AIDS in his relationship with Nikki? This inability to make the link between the facts of HIV transmission and personal risk is one of the core problems that HIV/AIDS education needs to address. [MG]

KOERTGE, RON. *The Arizona Kid*. Boston: Little, Brown, 1988. [Different editions have slightly different texts.] ISBN 0-7636-2542-6 (hardcover)

HIV/AIDS Content Scale: Accurate

HIV/AIDS Role in Story Scale: A subplot

Literary Quality Scale: Excellent

A pale redhead slick with sunblock wearing a vertically striped shirt to make himself look taller (this fools no one), sixteen-year-old Billy arrives from Bradleyville, Missouri, for a cowboy summer in Tucson, Arizona, with his gay Uncle Wes.

Billy has an inauspicious introduction to Tucson: He faints at the unaccustomed strength of the sun. But the summer improves for Billy in this often comic but deeply felt novel. He discovers that he is very good at working with horses at the racetrack and makes friends with his combat boot–clad coworker, Lew. Quirky characters abound, including Lew's survivalist father, Edgar, whose outrageous exploits provide some of the book's funniest moments. Coming of age in the time of HIV/AIDS, Billy happily casts off his virginity in safe sex with Cara Mae, the mercurial girl who exercises the horses. A horse race ends as it should, and two shady horse owners get their comeuppance in this very satisfying read.

In this book, HIV/AIDS is mostly a disease contracted by gay men. Although Wes does not have HIV/AIDS, many of his friends and associates do. We meet activists who campaign for education and understanding and the foul-mouthed thugs who attack them. Billy gets to know and admire Wes and his circle. He realizes that it is possible to have HIV/AIDS and still be healthy, like Luke, who "looks like an ad for vitamins" (p. 72). The stereotypes of gays and HIV/AIDS that Billy brings with him from Missouri are quickly dispelled as he grows into a caring, outspoken, accepting young man—a believably stronger version of the self-conscious boy whose first act in Tucson is to faint. [AYG]

LENNON, TOM. *When Love Comes to Town*. Dublin: O'Brien Press, 1993. ISBN 0-86278-361-5 (paperback)
HIV/AIDS Content Scale: Accurate
HIV/AIDS Role in Story Scale: A subplot
Literary Quality Scale: Very Good

Neil is popular at school and much loved at home, but he has never felt completely understood, seeing himself as a useless extra when invited to hang out with old friends who are part of twosomes ("the rhyming couplets"). Neil has known since the age of twelve that he is gay, and his anguished loneliness is palpable. Although he has been in love with a schoolmate, Ian, for years, Neil fears revealing his feelings. He frequently retreats into daydreams to avoid saying what he really thinks. Neil finally comes out to a close female friend, and then to his sister and her boyfriend, and plucks up the courage to seek out others like himself at a gay bar. He allows himself to be picked up by an older man of whom he is wary but who later saves his life when he is beaten by antigay thugs. At the bar, Neil also acquires a twenty-something lover named Shane and meets some outrageous gays and transsexuals who become his friends. Neil comes out to his Irish Catholic parents but discovers that he can maintain his relationship with them only by pretending that he does not sleep with men; however, the reader knows that Ian will be part of his future.

There are two characters with HIV/AIDS whose circumstances persuade Neil to come out to his parents. A woman on a radio call-in show describes how she discovered her son was gay, had AIDS, and then came home to die, making it clear that his sexual orientation and illness did not in any way affect her love for him. Daphne (really Eddie), one of Neil's new friends from the gay bar, is dying of AIDS. Neil and Shane visit him at his overcrowded flat in a rough Dublin neighborhood, where Neil is overwhelmed by the love that Daphne's mother lavishes on her son. Unfortunately Neil's parents are not as accepting. [AYG]

LEVY, MARILYN. *Rumors and Whispers*. New York: Fawcett Juniper/Ballantine Books, 1990. ISBN 0-449-70327-4 (paperback)
HIV/AIDS Content Scale: Accurate
HIV/AIDS Role in Story Scale: Central to plot
Literary Quality Scale: Good

Mr. Hill, shy Sarah Alexander's high school art teacher, is her hero. He makes her feel welcome in her new school and community and encourages her in her art. The other important new person in her life is David Light, her classmate and soon-to-be boyfriend. At home, however, things are not going well. Sarah hates Southern California and longs for her old life in Ohio. One day her father kicks her older brother, Doug, out of the house. Doug's crime is apparently so heinous that Mr. Alexander cannot even tell Sarah what it is, but she eventually learns that Doug is gay. When the news gets out that Mr. Hill is HIV positive and there is pressure from the community to dismiss him, Sarah and David want to fight to keep him in his job. For Sarah, this means choosing sides, because her father is intent on having Mr. Hill removed from the school. The school board decides to create an AIDS awareness program and apologizes to Mr. Hill. Sarah continues to stand up to her father by taking another course with Mr.

Hill and applying to an art school where she will be in the same city as David.

The picture of HIV/AIDS this book presents is that it is all around us and that attention must be paid to the epidemic. Sarah is first sensitized to the issue of HIV/AIDS by reading articles for a class in which she has been assigned to lead the discussion. She learns more from David and his father, a doctor and HIV/AIDS researcher. There is plenty of stigma directed at people with HIV/AIDS: Even Sarah, mistakenly thinking that Dr. Light has HIV/AIDS, briefly fears that kissing David has put her in danger simply because of his casual contact with his father. But stigma is also mitigated by the aptly (if not subtly) named Dr. Light, the voice of science and reason; a Christmas visit to his patients in the HIV/AIDS ward; and the appealing character of Jake, an HIV-positive resident who is a Light family friend. [AYG]

MCCLAIN, ELLEN JAFFE. *No Big Deal.* New York: Lodestar Books, 1994. ISBN 0-525-67483-7 (paperback)
HIV/AIDS Content Scale: Accurate
HIV/AIDS Role in Story Scale: A subplot
Literary Quality Scale: Good

Ninth grader Janice Green is a very bright student who tolerates her other teachers but adores Mr. Padovano, the only one who challenges her. It is "no big deal" to her if the rumors are true and Mr. P is gay. She gains an ally in her new best friend Holly, whose friendship is a great surprise and comfort to her because Holly is smart like Janice but pretty too. Janice, who is constantly harangued by her mother to lose weight, assumes that a pretty girl like Holly would not want to hang out with her. Although there is a realistic acknowledgment of the power of cliques and peer pressure, this novel tries to quash such stereotypes. Janice takes pains to protect Mr. P from the people (including her own mother) who are opposed to having a gay teacher in the school but is thwarted by her nemesis, Kevin Lynch, who she sees spray paint "Faggot" on Mr. P's car. Janice then blackmails him into joining the Academic All-Stars team that Mr. P coaches. Kevin turns out to be much smarter than he looks and (reluctantly) helps the team to a strong finish. But appearances are deceiving, and Janice starts to learn that the people around her have more complex motivations than she had thought.

The minimal HIV/AIDS content consists of incorrect rumors that Mr. P has the disease and a brief glimpse of someone who actually does have it—Kevin's gay older brother who lives in Greenwich Village. This connection provides the emotional background for Kevin's anger and actions. Janice thinks that having a gay brother should make Kevin empathetic toward Mr. P; however, Mr. P believes that Kevin resents him for being healthy when his brother is not. [AYG]

MCDANIEL, LURLENE. *Baby Alicia Is Dying*. New York: Bantam, 1993. ISBN 0-553-29605-1 (paperback)
HIV/AIDS Content Scale: Accurate
HIV/AIDS Role in Story Scale: Central to plot
Literary Quality Scale: Poor

As soon as teenager Desi Mitchell sets eyes on tiny Alicia at Childcare, a home for babies with HIV/AIDS whose teen mothers are drug addicts, she knows she must volunteer there. Desi pours all her pent-up affection onto Alicia because she does not get enough attention at home. Although Desi has accomplishments aplenty, it is her older sister Val, a freshman at college on a tennis scholarship, who has always been their mother's favorite. Mrs. Mitchell is critical of Desi's excessive devotion to her volunteer work, preferring that her daughter spend her time in more conventional activities. Although it may seem like Desi's mother is trying to protect Desi from contracting HIV/AIDS through casual contact, this is really a red herring. She does not want Desi to experience the death of a child she has grown to love, as happened when Desi's baby brother succumbed to crib death many years earlier. Alicia dies and Desi is devastated; however, in spite of Desi's resolve not to work at Childcare any longer, when she comes to visit she is drawn to Lucas, another baby who needs her.

The author acknowledges the staff and volunteers of Childkind in Atlanta, Georgia, which was likely the model for Childcare. The HIV/AIDS information in this novel is accurate, although labored. Much of it is presented in pamphletlike speeches from authority figures. The opening quote from the Gospel of Matthew places Desi's volunteering in the context of Christian charity, yet at least two main characters are anything but charitable. In a subplot, Desi's friend Brian describes how he felt betrayed when his uncle came out and told him that he had HIV/AIDS. Brian could not forgive his Uncle Mark for being gay, let alone sick, and Uncle Mark died alone. In another offstage incidence of HIV/AIDS, Val's fellow student Ted has the disease. Val cannot bring herself to talk to Ted because although he is healthy now, she sees Ted as a corpse-in-waiting. Although both Brian and Val are aware that their attitudes and actions are not admirable, Brian is still angry at his uncle, and Val does not plan to change her behavior toward Ted. [AYG]

MCDANIEL, LURLENE. *Sixteen and Dying*. (One Last Wish). New York: Bantam, 1992. ISBN 0-553-29932-8 (paperback)
HIV/AIDS Content Scale: Inaccurate
HIV/AIDS Role in Story Scale: Central to plot
Literary Quality Scale: Poor

As the result of a tainted blood transfusion received for injuries incurred in the same car accident that killed her mother, Anne Wingate is infected with the HIV virus. When Anne is diagnosed, an anonymous benefactor leaves a cashier's check for $100,000 under Anne's pillow while she sleeps at the hospital. She is urged to spend it as she wishes, so Anne chooses to forego treatment and spend the summer at a ranch, something she has always wanted to do. At the ranch, she meets Morgan, a darkly compelling boy who alternately angers and intrigues her. Anne makes other friends at the ranch and eventually settles in with Morgan, but she does not disclose her illness, afraid of potential consequences. When she becomes too ill to remain at the ranch, she does not say good-bye to Morgan, but he manages to find her back home in the city, where she finally discloses that she has AIDS. He in turn reveals his own struggles with a stigmatized disease, Huntington's, the illness that institutionalized his father. There is a chance that Morgan inherited Huntington's, but he is afraid to find out, so he refuses to have the test that would determine his status. Anne encourages Morgan to consider his future, going so far as to leave him enough money, after she dies, to get the Huntington's test. While Morgan's next actions are not revealed, there is a sense that Anne has had a lasting impact on his life and that he will likely get the test.

The overwhelming message about HIV in this novel is that it is a death sentence. Technical information about HIV is offered most often in thought form ("She knew AIDS wasn't contagious by kissing this way, but she was nervous anyway" [p. 101]) and is accurate in physical detail; however, according to the specialist Anne consults, "Women with AIDS are dying six times faster than men with AIDS. Once a woman is diagnosed with AIDS, her life expectancy is less than thirty weeks" (pp. 48–49). This information is simply untrue. Furthermore, Anne believes that contracting the disease gives everyone a reason to hate her; however, everyone who knows about Anne's illness treats her gently. A notable exception is the doctor who diagnoses Anne, grilling her in front of her father about her sex life and her use of injectable drugs, a third degree that is particularly absurd, given Anne's complete innocence and the fact that the car accident would have been part of her medical records. The mixed messages regarding the stigma of the disease end up being confusing. One can easily imagine a teen reader frightened that she might have HIV, but more frightened, as a result of having read this book, of going to a doctor with her fears, and thus potentially going undiagnosed. And while stigma related to HIV illness does exist and can be very damaging, the message and model provided here are not about coping but simply about avoiding anything that might potentially be unpleasant—do not tell anyone, hide, run away. [DC]

MAGUIRE, GREGORY. *Oasis*. New York: Clarion Books, 1996.
ISBN 0-395-67019-5 (hardcover)
HIV/AIDS Content Scale: Accurate
HIV/AIDS Role in Story Scale: Central to plot
Literary Quality Scale: Excellent

When his father dies unexpectedly, Hand is faced with more than just ordinary grieving. His mother returns, after having left the family (Hand, his father, and his sister, Vida) three years earlier, and Hand's feelings about her are very complicated—a mixture of hatred and longing that makes it almost impossible for Hand to cope with her presence. In addition, his Uncle Wolfgang, reviled by the extended family, has taken to corresponding with Hand, a fact that confuses Hand and adds a burden of guilt when he does not return the favor. When Nur and Vuffy, an Iranian immigrant and his small son, arrive at the Oasis (the motel that Hand's father once ran and that Hand and his mother have taken over) with a letter of approval from Hand's father to stay there, it seems just one more item in a long list of baffling occurrences. Hand takes their presence in stride with the coolness of an adolescent who simply does not know how to respond, but Vuffy's irrepressible spirit and obvious adoration of Hand and Nur's handiness around the motel work together to bring Hand out of the shell he has created for himself. And when his Uncle Wolfgang arrives to stay at the motel, little Vuffy acts as the bridge to Uncle Wolfgang that Hand lost when he lost his father, providing Hand the opportunity to finally bond with this complex and mysterious man.

Uncle Wolfgang is dying of AIDS when he comes to stay at the Oasis. As their relationship forms and deepens, Hand and Wolfgang talk about many things, AIDS among them. The topic of HIV is dealt with appropriately. It is an important but not all-encompassing issue in Hand's life, taking place among and within other family and acquaintance dynamics. Wolfgang is open about his disease without forcing information on unwilling parties, and information about HIV is skillfully woven in among natural interactions. [DC]

MANKELL, HENNING. *Playing with Fire*. Translated from Swedish by Anna Paterson. Crows Nest, NSW, Australia: Allen & Unwin, 2002. [First published as *Eldens Gåta* in Sweden by Rabén & Sjögren Bokförlag in 2001.] ISBN 1-86508-714-9 (paperback)

HIV/AIDS Content Scale: Accurate

HIV/AIDS Role in Story Scale: Central to plot

Literary Quality Scale: Excellent

Sofia and Rosa are sisters in Mozambique, Africa. Although their day-to-day life is one of hard work, minimal resources, and many other challenges, the sisters are close and share their burdens. Sofia, who lost her legs to a land mine as a child, takes up sewing and goes to school in hopes of having a better life one day. Rosa, the pretty one, helps their mother tend the fields and often goes out at night to dance and meet boys. While her mother worries that Rosa is pregnant, Rosa's tiredness turns out to be evidence that she is HIV positive.

Unlike other young adult novels that deal with HIV/AIDS in Africa, this story is less about the social ramifications of infection and more about the personal experience of one family dealing with a disease that threatens to "empty our villages" (p. 199). The depiction of Rosa's emotions as she weakens is starkly realistic, as is Sofia's budding womanhood in a context in which love is extremely dangerous, yet desired. Infection with HIV in this circumstance is most likely to be a death sentence, as the characters know that money for medicines necessary to extend the life of the infected is beyond their reach. [MG]

MIKLOWITZ, GLORIA D. *Good-Bye Tomorrow.* New York: Delacorte Press, 1987. ISBN 0-385-29562-6 (hardcover)
HIV/AIDS Content Scale: Accurate
HIV/AIDS Role in Story Scale: Central to plot
Literary Quality Scale: Good

Seventeen-year-old Alex Weiss is a popular guy with a bright future: He has a girlfriend, a job, a regular spot on the high school swim team, and plans for college. He is devastated when he is diagnosed with ARC (AIDS-related complex), caused by the unscreened blood transfusions that saved his life after a car accident several years earlier. For Alex, the worst part of it is the fear that he may have inadvertently infected his girlfriend, Shannon, through unprotected sex. (Ironically, Shannon had gone on the pill to prevent pregnancy, but she and Alex were not as careful about using condoms to prevent disease.) The story is told by three first-person narrators: Alex, Shannon, and Alex's fifteen-year-old sister, Christy. This narrative device capitalizes on the intimacy of the first person. At the same time, it allows suspense to build as Shannon and Christy try to discover why Alex is so standoffish. Finally, it reveals their secret thoughts and anxieties about dealing with the impending public knowledge of Alex's illness.

There is a lot of AIDS stigma in this novel and just a few people who support Alex. Even his sister, who has read clippings about the disease and knows better, has qualms about casual contact with him. Shannon is naturally on edge until she tests negative and even then has to force herself to maintain her friendship with Alex in spite of her unabated feelings for him. Both Christy and Shannon experience a mixture of loyalty, love, embarrassment, shame, and, ultimately, courage, in confronting their admittedly unreasonable fears. The adults in charge vary in their reactions. Although the swim team coach is supportive, the principal does not want any trouble with parents objecting to Alex's presence at school and requires that Alex take "sick leave," which is tantamount to suspension. Crusty Dr. Hoff is perhaps the most helpful, dispensing accurate information as well as good advice. Since this is one of the earliest novels dealing with HIV/AIDS, methods of diagnosis and treatment have changed. Although Alex does not have full-blown AIDS, he urges Shannon to go out with other people, seeing no future for them as a couple, or for himself: "good-bye tomorrow" indeed. [AYG]

MINCHIN, ADELE. *The Beat Goes On*. New York: Simon & Schuster, 2004. [First published in Great Britain by Livewire Books, the Women's Press Limited, in 2001.] ISBN 0-689-86611-9 (hardcover)

HIV/AIDS Content Scale: Accurate
HIV/AIDS Role in Story Scale: Central to plot
Literary Quality Scale: Very good

Fifteen-year-old Leyla's cousin Emma confides that she is HIV positive and asks Leyla to keep her secret. As hard as it is to do this and work through her own emotional reaction to her cousin's illness, Leyla helps Emma as best she can. She does so by listening to her fears, volunteering at Emma's support center, and not telling her parents about Emma's condition. Emma and her mother both fear what will happen if people find out, and there are many examples in the book of the social isolation and even violence families affected by HIV/AIDS experience. Leyla's parents eventually do find out about Emma's condition, deepening the rift between Leyla's and Emma's mothers. Emma and her mother move away, and only when Emma is hospitalized is Leyla able to render some compassion out of her own mother for her own suffering, if not that of her cousin and aunt.

Some of the strong points of this story are how honest it is about adolescent sexuality and how it models the need to negotiate safer sex practices. Another strength is its depiction of the emotional effect of the disease on those who have it as well as on their family and friends. Set in England, the narrative takes some getting used to for the American ear, but many will find the difference in word use interesting and at times delightful. For instance, at one point in the story Leyla's boyfriend compliments her by noting how "really sorted" (p. 111) she is. On the downside, while the progression of HIV infection varies among individuals, informed readers will question how a teenager infected through vertical transmission, in what must have been the early days of the AIDS epidemic, has managed to survive and stay healthy, while Emma, with the benefit of current medicine, suffers a sharp decline over the course of a year. [MG]

MITCHELL, NANCY. *Raging Skies*. Changing Earth Trilogy, Book Two. Fremont, CA: Lightstream Publications, 1999. ISBN 1-892713-01-2 (paperback)

HIV/AIDS Content Scale: Accurate

HIV/AIDS Role in Story Scale: A subplot

Literary Quality Scale: Poor

It is 2018 in the East Bay area, and wheelchair-bound teen Jenny Powers and her friends and family must cope with two separate natural disasters: a newly active volcano and flooding due to an earthquake-damaged reservoir. As if this were not enough, the book has a frame story involving male power brokers and scientists who plan to control the burgeoning population with a new virus that will affect female fertility. Incidentally, Jenny's friend Amelia has contracted HIV from a boyfriend (she is not sure which one) and has no compunction about spreading it around. This surprisingly unimaginative middle book in the Changing Earth science fiction trilogy suffers from superficial emotion, boring action scenes, and execrable writing. The author seems much more interested in disaster planning than character development, but even the scenes in which the students quickly organize relief efforts are completely unrealistic.

There is little HIV/AIDS-related content. Since the book is set in the future, it would have been reasonable to propose new treatments or even a cure, but the author does not posit any new developments in HIV/AIDS research. Jenny thinks that keeping a confidence—that Amelia is HIV positive—outweighs the serious public health consequences. Jenny does attempt to get the doctor at the high school health clinic to intervene, but the solution they come up with, that is to ask the sister of Amelia's prospective boyfriend to persuade him to use a condom, without mentioning HIV/AIDS, is lame. [AYG]

MOORE, STEPHANIE PERRY. *Laurel Shadrach Series 1: Purity Reigns.* Chicago: Moody Press, 2002. ISBN 0-8024-4035-5 (paperback)
HIV/AIDS Content Scale: Accurate
HIV/AIDS Role in Story Scale: Mentioned in passing
Literary Quality Scale: Poor

Laurel Shadrach expects her senior year at college in Conyers, Georgia, to be perfect: She is popular, has a handsome boyfriend named Branson, and has an excellent chance of getting a gymnastics scholarship to college. Instead of being able to glory in all this, however, she falls out with her friends, breaks up (yet again) with Branson, and sprains her ankle during a gymnastics practice. When things get tough for her (or anyone else), Laurel relies on her evangelical Christian faith to see her (and them) through. Branson constantly pressures Laurel to have sex with him. Although she is tempted, she remains steadfast, precipitating the breakup. Her best friend Brittany betrays her by having a sexual relationship with Branson. Laurel finds a more suitable, more handsome boyfriend, Foster, who, like her, wants to date "God's way" (p. 172), but bad boy Branson is always a temptation in the wings.

The HIV/AIDS content is very limited. Laurel finds out that Brittany's ex-boyfriend, Justin, is HIV positive. The reader is left wondering whether Brittany, and therefore Branson, has been infected, too. [AYG]

MOORE, STEPHANIE PERRY. *Laurel Shadrach Series 2: Totally Free.* Chicago: Moody Press, 2002. ISBN 0-8024-4036-3 (paperback)
HIV/AIDS Content Scale: Accurate
HIV/AIDS Role in Story Scale: A subplot
Literary Quality Scale: Poor

Laurel is a Christian girl who uses her faith to deal with every aspect of her life, from coping with alcoholism among her family and friends to dealing with day-to-day problems in her social life. Nonetheless, Laurel keeps bad company, keeps secrets from her parents, drinks, pits her suitors against each other, and makes the wrong choice at every turn. Meanwhile, her best friend Brittany is able to steal Laurel's boyfriend because she is sexually active.

Later, Brittany learns that an old boyfriend has AIDS and subsequently tests positive for HIV herself. This news worries Laurel's ex-beau, who fears he may have HIV, too. This motivates him to seek emotional support and reconciliation with Laurel.

The HIV/AIDS content in this story is fairly minimal but problematic. When Brittany goes to the clinic to hear the results of her HIV test, the doctor knocks her out with sedatives because she seems upset. He then shares her diagnosis with Laurel and calls Brittany's parents without consulting her. This scenario is unfortunate, for it may reinforce young people's fears about being tested and leave them with the impression that they have no right to privacy and confidentiality in medical situations. All told, HIV/AIDS is just another micro drama in Laurel's life that really does not affect her all that much. Little is offered about the realities of dealing with HIV infection from any standpoint. [MG]

MOORE, STEPHANIE PERRY. *Laurel Shadrach Series 3: Equally Yoked*. Chicago: Moody Publishers, 2003. ISBN 0-8024-4037-1 (paperback)

HIV/AIDS Content Scale: Accurate
HIV/AIDS Role in Story Scale: Mentioned in passing
Literary Quality Scale: Poor

Laurel's senior year in high school is coming to an end, and her life continues on its dramatic and chaotic trajectory. Although she professes a deep faith and trust in God and never hesitates to create opportunities for both public and private expressions of this faith (winning souls to God is a running theme throughout the series), her actions and choices repeatedly belie whatever impulse to integrity she might possess. Racism is a primary issue in this installment of the series, and it is treated in a predictably melodramatic and inauthentic manner. While racism surely does exist in real life, it is typically rather more subtle in its manifestation than in this series of novels.

Brittany, who is HIV positive, is still a part of Laurel's life, but apart from a bit of whining on Brittany's part, her HIV status is a completely peripheral issue. The drama of discovery/diagnosis has already been addressed, and it is too early for the drama of HIV-related illness, given Brittany's youth and health and the early detection of the HIV. Rather than addressing the very real issues surrounding being a teen with HIV, the author has made

Brittany's whining superficial, and used it only as an opportunity for Laurel to win her friend "back" to Christ. [DC]

MOORE, STEPHANIE PERRY. *Laurel Shadrach Series 4: Absolutely Worthy*. Chicago: Moody Publishers, 2003. ISBN 0-8024-4038-X (paperback)

HIV/AIDS Content Scale: Accurate
HIV/AIDS Role in Story Scale: Mentioned in passing
Literary Quality Scale: Poor

Laurel Shadrach is now a college freshman and coping with many temptations that distract her from being what she considers a good Christian. She misses out on a prestigious gymnastics scholarship due to a sprained ankle but is given an opportunity to compete for a walk-on spot on the team; however, she pledges a sorority and is, improbably, unanimously elected as the pledge class president. This responsibility comes at the expense of gymnastics practice. She just cannot shake her attraction to her ex-boyfriend from high school, Branson, who has inconveniently also been accepted to the University of Georgia. Since Branson had long been pressuring her to have sex and she had broken off the relationship because she was not ready, it is hard to maintain any serious sympathy for her. As is usual in this series, there is a lot of plot. In addition to sports, sororities, and boyfriends, Laurel copes with separation from her family, learns to get along with her black roommate, her upwardly mobile suitemate, and deals with a suicide attempt by another suitemate and the murder of a student from her dorm. Everything is resolved by Laurel putting herself in God's hands and witnessing to others. The writing is unsophisticated and predictable. The treatment of racism borders on offensive. Character development is limited. One selfish girlfriend (Jewels) looks and sounds very much like another (Brittany).

Laurel's HIV-positive friend, Brittany, makes brief appearances at the beginning and the end of the book. The information provided about HIV/AIDS is minimal and not always presented clearly. For example, while maintaining a positive attitude is important to managing Brittany's disease, to do this "so the cells won't take over" (p. 185) suggests a murky understanding of how T cells operate. Laurel and Brittany's other best friend, Meagan, meanwhile sleeps with two different guys within a very short time and becomes pregnant and is unsure which one is the father of her child. It might perhaps be argued that teen hormones and lack of judgment could lead Meagan to sleep with one boy without protection, even though her best friend has HIV, but it defies all credibility that she would sleep with two boys she did not really know, within such a short time of each other, and without any form of protection at all. [AYG/DC]

MOORE, STEPHANIE PERRY. *Laurel Shadrach Series 5: Finally Sure.* Chicago: Moody Publishers, 2004. ISBN 0-8024-4039-8 (paperback)

HIV/AIDS Content Scale: Accurate

HIV/AIDS Role in Story Scale: Mentioned in passing

Literary Quality Scale: Poor

The predominant themes of this installment in the Laurel Shadrach series are the importance of witnessing and the threat of eternal separation from God for those who have not been saved. During the spring semester at the University of Georgia, Laurel becomes increasingly in touch with how important her religious convictions are to her as she replaces the possibility of competing on an Olympic-level gymnastics team with cheerleading, becomes more involved with her sorority, and builds a relationship with a mysterious young man in the library. Laurel also continues to be unreliable, selfish, given to bouts of violence and drinking, and still desires a relationship with her old boyfriend.

Laurel's HIV-positive friend Brittany has given up promiscuity, is taking care of her health, and is finally following the Lord. She has little part in the day-to-day drama of Laurel's life, as she too is away at school. Brittany's main value for Laurel is the didactic tale she provides when one of Laurel's sorority sisters confides that she is thinking about having sex. There are no other characters in this story who are dealing with HIV/AIDS in any respect, and the narrative does not provide any other information about how HIV/AIDS might affect the lives of students at college. For readers who do not share the religious orientation of the characters in this story, the heavily didactic and one-sided point of view may prove tiresome. For others, main character Laurel will seem an unlikable person whose concerns and self-centeredness limit her ability for growth. [MG]

NELSON, THERESA. *Earthshine.* New York: Orchard Books, 1994. ISBN 0-531-06867-6 (hardcover)
HIV/AIDS Content Scale: Accurate
HIV/AIDS Role in Story Scale: Central to plot
Literary Quality Scale: Excellent

Slim's parents are divorced. Because living with her mother means she has to move frequently, never allowing her to set down roots, Slim has chosen to live with her father Mack and his partner Larry. Mack is an actor, funny and clever, and HIV positive. Slim attends a support group of kids who are living with somebody who has AIDS, and it is here that she meets Isaiah. Isaiah's father died of AIDS, and his pregnant mother is HIV positive. In spite of these circumstances, or perhaps because of them, Isaiah has a magical outlook on life. He believes alternately in the falsity of death and in a miracle cure for HIV that requires a challenging, multifamily quest through the mountains to acquire "Dragon Tears"—an elixir said to cure any illness. The use of humor throughout the novel, in exposition and as a coping mechanism used by the characters in times of crisis, makes the subject matter not only bearable but even transforming. Here, the loss experienced as a result of Mack's death is balanced by the birth of Isaiah's baby sister, Halley, who is free of HIV infection. Even the spreading of Mack's ashes, in a place of incongruous (and thus perfect) spiritual significance, is infused with the gentle humor and acceptance characterized by the novel as a whole.

This novel is populated with characters depicted in various stages of HIV infection, from ill and dying to seemingly healthy. The information provided never feels preachy or didactic, rather it is fitted seamlessly into the narrative. And while the situations depicted are often quite dark and disturbing (for example, a carnival that is interrupted when skinheads start throwing glass bottles and shouting hateful messages), humor and resilience triumph in the end. [DC]

NOLAN, HAN. *Born Blue.* New York: Harcourt, 2001. ISBN 0-15-201916-2 (hardcover)
HIV/AIDS Content Scale: Accurate
HIV/AIDS Role in Story Scale: A subplot
Literary Quality Scale: Excellent

The core of Janie's identity is her ability to sing, and her driving ambition is to be an Ella Fitzgerald, Sarah Vaughn, Etta James, or Billie Holiday. It is not surprising that she would cling to the blues as a young child, listening to their tapes on a Fisher Price tape player. Unwanted, neglected, given away by her mother as part of a drug deal, and fending for herself by the age of twelve, her voice and her desire to sing drive her forward, while her damaging past dooms her to repeat a pattern of using and then driving away those who care enough to try to help her. The amazing strength of this novel is in the voice it gives to Janie, who finds her voice but cannot escape a life propelled by betrayal.

At the age of sixteen, after an unwanted pregnancy, some success with her music, and burning every bridge she has, Janie looks up her heroin-addicted mother and finds that Mama Linda is dying of AIDS. Terrified, she turns to run but ends up staying a few months until her mother passes away. During this time, she learns to overcome many unwarranted fears about catching the disease, learns a little more about her past, and develops some insight about how similar she is to her mother. This is not enough to tame our hero, however, who characteristically steals some money and slips out on the well-meaning neighbor to take to the road again. This grippingly realistic portrayal puts the reader inside the experience of an abandoned and abused child growing up with a single dream. [MG]

PAULSEN, GARY. *The Car*. Orlando, FL: Harcourt Brace & Company, 1994. ISBN 0-15-292878-2 (hardcover)
HIV/AIDS Content Scale: Accurate
HIV/AIDS Role in Story Scale: Mentioned in passing
Literary Quality Scale: Good

Terry finds himself on his own when his divorcing parents abandon him. While he waits for one of them to come back, he passes the time working on a car kit left in the garage. Somewhat implausibly Terry is able to put the car together and then manages to teach himself to drive in order to get to his uncle, who lives on the other side of the country. These plans almost immediately go off course when he picks up a war vet named Waylon and starts out on a cross-country journey that is part history, part philosophy, and part self-discovery. After several eye-opening events, Waylon and his friends get into a fight with some bikers and violence ensues. There is going to be a showdown, and Waylon talks Terry into taking off in the car. Terry hits the road but is uncertain as he considers whether he wants to abandon his friends to track down an uncle he barely knows.

In one of several adventures, Terry, Waylon, and his friends stop to see Mary, a prostitute Waylon knew when he was in the army. They learn that she died of AIDS and are told that this should be expected, given the nature of her work. The overt moral is that Mary should not be judged for her profession or fate, as she was a good person who gave Waylon the strength he needed to stay in the army when he wanted to desert. [MG]

PECK, RICHARD. *The Last Safe Place on Earth.* New York: Delacorte Press, 1995. ISBN 0-385-32052-3 (hardcover)
HIV/AIDS Content Scale: Accurate
HIV/AIDS Role in Story Scale: Mentioned in passing
Literary Quality Scale: Excellent

Todd has a great family. They live in the best part of town, with the best schools, the best neighbors, and the best opportunities. Then one night Laurel shows up to babysit Todd's little sister, and Todd's world is turned upside down. Laurel is beautiful—she's perfect, she's mysterious—everything Todd could want, but Laurel's world is complicated by an intolerant and fanatic religious orientation, a younger brother who constantly ups the ante in testing the boundaries of the law, and parents who are by turns abusive and absent. Laurel finds some sort of solace in the strictures of her family's religious beliefs; but when she attempts to indoctrinate Todd's little sister using fear tactics, Todd's family circles the wagons. And when books and activities are challenged at Todd's school, it turns out this same religious sect is behind most of the complaints, and Todd eventually discovers that the very worst sort of censorship is that you bring on yourself, by choosing not to be aware.

The HIV content in this novel is barely there; in fact, it is its absence that is at issue here, the numbers of people who refuse to see HIV as an important issue and worthy of their time and attention. The one character we encounter who has AIDS is a speaker at an event that almost no one attends. All we know about her or her experience is that she has AIDS. As a social commentary on the general public response, this novel is excellent; however, it understandably offers little in the way of facts about the disease. [DC]

PECK, RICHARD. *Strays Like Us.* New York: Puffin Books, 1998. ISBN 0-8037-2291-5 (hardcover)
HIV/AIDS Content Scale: Accurate
HIV/AIDS Role in Story Scale: A subplot
Literary Quality Scale: Very good

Molly has been sent to live with her Aunt Fay while her mother is hospitalized for drug addiction. She resists her neighbor Will's attempts to befriend her, certain that her mother will return soon, but days turn into weeks and the summer comes to an end. Molly remains a detached participant at her new school but finds unexpected companionship in a homeschooled girl, Tracy Pringle, and a cantankerous home patient of Aunt Fay's, Mrs. Voorhees. And while her relationship with Will is still distant and uncertain, the two are brought together when Molly learns that Fay has secretly been providing nursing care to Will's father, who has AIDS. When her mother is arrested for dealing drugs, Molly is given the opportunity to take root where she is, and she discovers family in the most unlikely of places.

HIV plays a very minor role in this story, as does, in fact, Will's father, the one character infected with HIV. The information provided is accurate enough, there is just very little to go on. The fear of stigma is potent for both Will and Molly but is perhaps overstated, given the circumstances. In a literary sense, the fact that Will's father remains a secret almost until his death, and that he only figures in the third person, heightens the story's mystery and adds to its flavor. Informationally, however, it fails to shed much light on the facts and issues surrounding infection with HIV. [DC]

PIKE, CHRISTOPHER. *The Last Vampire.* New York: Archway Paperbacks, 1994. ISBN 0-671-87264-8 (paperback)
HIV/AIDS Content Scale: Inaccurate (vampirism)
HIV/AIDS Role in Story Scale: A subplot
Literary Quality Scale: Good

Alisa Pern may be more than 5,000 years old, yet her youth, beauty, and attitude clearly mark her as a case of arrested development. Her ennui and her belief in her own infallibility also work to allow the reader to get that she is really a member of this book's intended audience. What happens to an eighteen-year-old who can never die? Over the course of the novel the reader hears about Alisa's early life in India, how she becomes a vampire, and why she is being tracked by the only other vampire left on the planet. As she enlists the help of local high schoolers in her effort to avoid being killed, we learn that her would-be biographer, Seymour, has full-blown AIDS.

This is the only work in which a cure for HIV/AIDS is posited. One of the perks of vampirism is possession of a super immune system, which is why vampires do not get sick from any of the blood they drink. Alisa is able to cure Seymour by replacing his blood with her own—not enough to turn him into a vampire, just enough to save him. This ensures that even if she turns out to be unsuccessful in her final fight, her story will be told. [MG]

PIKE, CHRISTOPHER. *The Midnight Club*. New York: Archway Paperbacks, 1994. ISBN 0-671-87263-X (paperback)
HIV/AIDS Content Scale: Accurate
HIV/AIDS Role in Story Scale: A subplot
Literary Quality Scale: Good

Ilonka Pawluk lives in a hospice for terminally ill teens. She and four friends form a storytelling support group that meets at midnight. Ilonka, her roommate Anya, Kevin, Spence, and Sandra enjoy the camaraderie and learn more about one another through their stories, made-up tales that reflect aspects of their real lives. Ilonka recounts stories of what she believes to be her past lives, all revolving around an Eastern mystical figure called the Master and featuring someone resembling Kevin, with whom she is in love. Kevin shares Ilonka's feelings, although he already has a girlfriend. Ilonka remorselessly dispatches the competition by telling Kevin's girlfriend, who is in denial about Kevin's fate, the truth of his impending death. This is ironic because Ilonka has not fully accepted that she herself is dying. In the end, everyone is forgiven for the terrible things they have done.

Teresa, a character in Kevin's story, is diagnosed with HIV/AIDS. At the end of her life she is briefly reunited with Herme, her former lover whom she betrayed. Herme is an angel-turned-mortal, a gifted painter, the muse of the great Renaissance artists, who later in life becomes a doctor, which is how he meets up with Teresa again. In an equally dramatic real-life deathbed confession, Spence tells Ilonka that he killed his lover, Carl, by inadvertently passing on the HIV virus to him, and that Spence's brain tumor is an AIDS-related complication. [AYG]

PINSKER, JUDITH. *Robin's Diary*. Radnor, PA: ABC Daytime Press/Chilton Book Company, 1995. [Based on the story by Claire Labine.] ISBN 0-8019-8775-X (paperback)
HIV/AIDS Content Scale: Accurate
HIV/AIDS Role in Story Scale: Central to plot
Literary Quality Scale: Good

Based on the ABC daytime drama *General Hospital*, this is the personal diary of high school student Robin Scorpio, detailing her coming-of-age story as she falls in love with and then loses Michael "Stone" Cates to AIDS. Both characters suffered the loss of their parents early in life, and Robin is being raised by her loving uncle, while Stone has had to make do for himself living on the streets of New York. During this time, Stone had unprotected sex with several partners, including one young woman who used drugs. Although he tested negative before he met Robin, he has AIDS and infects her when she starts taking birth control pills and they stop using condoms, thinking they only needed to worry about pregnancy.

While the plot development cannot help but reveal the "soap opera" nature of the original story, the insights provided into Robin's developing feelings for and loyalty to Stone as well as the detail concerning the development, treatment, and course of AIDS is realistic and informing. One cannot help but develop empathy and even respect for Robin, who demonstrates a high level of compassion and manages a tragic situation in an exemplary fashion. The consequences of unprotected sex are clear here, as is the necessity for empathy and support between friends and family and from society as well. [MG]

PLUM-UCCI, CAROL. *What Happened to Lani Garver*. Orlando, FL: Harcourt, 2002. ISBN 0-15-216813-3 (hardcover)
HIV/AIDS Content Scale: Accurate
HIV/AIDS Role in Story Scale: Mentioned in passing
Literary Quality Scale: Excellent

This book is fast paced, intricate, mysterious. The question of who Lani Garver is and the ultimate fate of a character who rejects characterization lingers in the reader's memory long after the last page. What we do know is that Lani tends to bring out both the best and the worst in people, mainly by being willing to recognize and speak the truth. Lani is a life-changing agent in Claire's life, and the subtheme of survival works its way through the lives of several characters who are dealing with extreme challenges, everything from anorexia and alcoholism to leukemia and HIV/AIDS. It is the struggle against peer pressure and society's rejection of difference that provides the main tension for Claire. She desperately, but at times unknowingly, needs to find a way to be in the world that will allow her to maintain her health and individuality. With Lani's help she gets there. What happens to Lani is left to the reader to consider.

The fact that the characters with HIV/AIDS play only a minor part in the story limits the amount of HIV/AIDS-related information expressed; however, there is a clear sense that characters facing life-threatening circumstances can continue to live useful, creative lives and that small-mindedness has its own consequences in the world. [MG]

PORTE, BARBARA ANN. *Something Terrible Happened.* New York: Orchard Books, 1994. ISBN 0-531-06869-2 (hardcover)
HIV/AIDS Content Scale: Accurate
HIV/AIDS Role in Story Scale: A subplot
Literary Quality Scale: Passable

Gillian has spent most of her young life living with her mother and grandmother in a comfortable apartment in New York City. Gillian's father died when she was very small, and all she really remembers about him was that he was white and didn't mind that her mother was not. Gillian's family is ambitious, as evidenced by her mother's teaching and acting careers and the fact that her grandmother is in training to run a marathon. But when Gillian's mother falls terribly ill, the solution Gillian's grandmother comes up with seems like giving up: She sends Gillian to live with her father's brother, whom she has never met and who does not share the West Indian culture in which Gillian was raised. Gillian is understandably resentful at first, but she learns to adapt, forming friendships with her new family even as she misses her grandmother and mourns her mother's death. The unidentified narrator claims to be a school friend of Gillian's grandmother, and the apparent implication is that this makes her somehow intimate with the entire family. The reader is not shown this relationship, however, but only told it exists, which makes the narration jarring and confusing.

It is made clear from the start that to be diagnosed with AIDS is to be given a death sentence. When Gillian's mother finds out she is HIV positive, she ignores the treatments prescribed by doctors, seeking alternative treatments instead, no matter how off the wall they may be. One such attempt takes her to Florida, where the illness worsens and she and Gillian are left homeless and penniless—it is clear that the HIV has affected both her body and her mind. [DC]

RIVERS, KAREN. *Dream Water*. Custer, WA: Orca Book Publishers, 1999. [Canadian editorial office in Victoria, BC.] ISBN 1-55143-160-2 (hardcover)

HIV/AIDS Content Scale: Accurate

HIV/AIDS Role in Story Scale: A subplot

Literary Quality Scale: Poor

Several children witness the death of a trainer in a pool of killer whales, and each finds their own way to cope. Cassie has relegated the experience to nightmares, while Holden tries to express it in painting. When Cassie starts going to dance school she loses touch with Holden and focuses obsessively on earning the lead in an upcoming major production. In the meantime, Holden is becoming increasingly dependent on alcohol. Then Holden's mother returns home, sick with AIDS, after having abandoned the family years earlier; and Cassie encounters a teacher at her school who is passionate about whales' rights. These encounters become the unlikely catalysts that propel the two, now teenagers, toward finally healing from their shared childhood trauma.

While there is a character featured who has AIDS, her presence is largely peripheral. She comes into the story thin and old looking; she gets pneumonia and dies—a junkie who paid her dues. The symptoms and illness are not inaccurate, they are just barely there. In fact, even the protagonists' struggles with the aftermath of witnessing a violent death are peripheral to the author's Save the Whales agenda, and even that is not pieced together effectively. [DC]

ROPER, GAYLE. *The Case of the Missing Melody.* East Edge Mysteries, No. 4. Elgin, IL: Chariot Books/David C. Cook Publishing Co., 1993. ISBN 1-55513-702-4 (paperback)
HIV/AIDS Content Scale: Accurate
HIV/AIDS Role in Story Scale: A subplot
Literary Quality Scale: Passable

Eleven-year-old Charlie's alcoholic mother has abandoned her one time too many. Now her mother is going off to California with a new boyfriend and does not want Charlie to come along. Charlie has found a good home with her Christian foster parents, the Andersons, where she gets the love, attention, and structure she has been lacking. However, it is Melody, the baby the Andersons have taken in because Melody's mother, an HIV-positive crack addict, cannot care for her, with whom she bonds most closely. Melody is kidnapped when she is in Charlie's care, and, devastated, Charlie resolves to find her and bring her home. Charlie's friends from church, the girls in the Kids Care Club, are as eager to help Charlie as they are to rescue Melody. The kidnapper turns out to be Melody's teenage aunt, whose misguided plan to return Melody to her mother backfires when Charlie and her friends intervene. Charlie is then invited to join the club.

When Melody is diagnosed with HIV, Charlie's devotion to her never wavers. Charlie carefully follows Mrs. Anderson's instructions on how to safely handle the baby, so she does not feel that she is in the slightest danger of contracting the disease herself. Mrs. Anderson predicts that some of the church members will reject Melody out of fear, but in this book that does not happen. [AYG]

ROPER, GAYLE. *The Mystery of the Poison Pen.* East Edge Mysteries, No. 5. Elgin, IL: Chariot Books/David C. Cook Publishing Co., 1994. ISBN 0-7814-1507-1 (paperback)
HIV/AIDS Content Scale: Inaccurate
HIV/AIDS Role in Story Scale: Central to plot
Literary Quality Scale: Poor

A foster family in Alysha's church has just found out that the baby they are taking care of is HIV positive. This news has required some rethinking about this family's participation in the congregation. While the overt message from the church elders and the congregation is that we need to be nice to these people, new rules are instituted that apply only to them. For instance, baby Melody can no longer be in the nursery with the other children, and her foster mother must sit outside the sanctuary with Melody if she wants to attend services; however, one member of the congregation does not want Melody at church at all and begins leaving threatening messages, such as "Get that kid out of here before she kills someone! I'm warning you!" (p. 16). Alysha decides that she needs to figure out who is sending these notes and begins collecting clues.

The misinformation about the risks of HIV infection and the attitude of the congregation toward Melody and her foster family are shocking. When it is determined that it is not safe for Melody to be with the other children, the Sunday school teacher—a nurse—enlists a group of twelve-year-old girls to clean the nursery and the toys to make it safe for the little ones. The logic behind this is mindboggling. If there really is some danger here, why are children being asked to remove the risk with sudsy water? Adults and others who voice their fears about HIV are considered to be behaving inappropriately. At the same time, the determination of the parishioners to only use compassionate words is undercut by the not-so-subtle accommodations that allow Melody and her family to come to church but also openly stigmatize them for reasons that do not reflect reasonable fears of transmission. [MG]

ST. JOHN, CHARLOTTE. *Red Hair Three.* New York: Fawcett Juniper, 1992. ISBN 0-449-70406-8 (paperback)
HIV/AIDS Content Scale: Accurate
HIV/AIDS Role in Story Scale: Central to plot
Literary Quality Scale: Passable

Identical twins, separated when young and reunited on school vacations at the beach in Florida, fall in love with boys who do not love them and learn the perils of early sexuality. Elaine loves nasty college boy Dean, who is dying of AIDS. Lucky for her, she did not have sex with him, even though he broke up with her because she would not give in. Now, although he confides that he does not love her, was highly promiscuous, and took performance-enhancing drugs, she finds herself more drawn to him than ever. Her love for him is such that she chooses to spend her summer vacation by his side as his health deteriorates. Dean lets Elaine keep him company but shows little insight and is selfish and ugly to the end. Twin Emily, on the other hand, broke up with Kyle and hardly looked back until she learned that her dumping him really did not affect him much at all. Now that he is heartbroken over Michelle, Emily finds she wants him after all. As if that were not reason enough to give a young girl pause, Nita and Susannah, two minor characters in the story, pay the price of early sexuality by becoming pregnant. Nita's parents are able to help her make the decision to terminate her pregnancy. Susannah's wealthy parents talk her into marrying Broderick, who will live in a room far on the other side of the mansion, while the housekeeper raises the baby. How do Elaine and Emily respond to all of this? Elaine already has a line on some hunky Hollywood notables, and a fall vacation in California is in sight.

The facts about HIV/AIDS presented in this novel are accurate; however, once diagnosed, Dean's health declines rapidly. He learns he is HIV positive in December, and before summer's end he is gone. It is as though the news itself was enough to do him in. [MG]

SANCHEZ, ALEX. *The God Box.* New York: Simon & Schuster Books for Young Readers, 2007. ISBN-10 1-4169-0899-4 (hardcover)

HIV/AIDS Content Scale: Accurate

HIV/AIDS Role in Story Scale: Mentioned in passing

Literary Quality Scale: Good

Paul suspects that he may be gay, but his thoughts and inclinations clearly go against his religion and are not acceptable in the small Texas town where he lives. Paul is able to sublimate most of his feelings until a new student, Manuel, shows up at school. Manuel is openly gay, a Christian, and interested in developing a relationship with Paul. Paul finds Manuel both compelling and threatening. In response, Paul begins to work through whether he can be his true self and still be loved by God, family, and friends.

When Paul goes to his pastor for help, he refers him to an organization that claims it can help him stay "straight." Paul is visited by an "exgay" man, Eric, who talks at length about his previous gay lifestyle, which he feels he has overcome; however, Paul is not convinced by Eric's story. In his exploits, Eric experienced a terrible scare when he learned that a man he had unprotected sex with was HIV positive. This is the only mention of HIV/AIDS in this story, which is primarily concerned with reconciling homosexuality with biblical teachings. [MG]

SANCHEZ, ALEX. *Rainbow Boys*. New York: Simon & Schuster, 2001. ISBN 0-689-85770-5 (paperback)
HIV/AIDS Content Scale: Accurate
HIV/AIDS Role in Story Scale: A subplot
Literary Quality Scale: Good

The first book in the Rainbow Boys trilogy is a romance novel oriented to the internal conflicts, social issues, and identity development of three gay high school seniors. Each of these characters traverses, in his own way, the challenge of being truthful about his sexual orientation and the emotional vicissitudes of first love and first sexual experiences. While the young men have to deal with homophobia and lack of understanding on the part of adults and peers, overall Whitman High and the surrounding community is a very welcoming one. When confronted with the existence of gay and lesbian students, the community, for the most part, makes space for them as though their previous marginalization was an unintended faux pas. How much easier life would be for many if acceptance were always so easily achieved.

The difficulties of coming of age in the time of HIV/AIDS are dealt with on a personal level, revealing how complicated "staying safe" can be. The story is realistic in portraying characters who fail to follow safer sex practices and showing how hard it can be to deal with issues of HIV status in dating relationships. The story is also successful in stressing the need for communication between people and the strength that self-esteem and social support can bring young people working through new feelings on their way to adulthood and a healthy sense of self. [MG]

SANCHEZ, ALEX. *Rainbow High*. New York: Simon Pulse, 2003. ISBN 0-689-85477-3 (hardcover)
HIV/AIDS Content Scale: Accurate
HIV/AIDS Role in Story Scale: A subplot
Literary Quality Scale: Good

In the second installment in the Rainbow Boys series, gay friends Kyle, Jason, and Nelson are high school seniors who have helped set up the new Gay-Straight Alliance to fight homophobia in their suburban Washington, D.C., school. Swimmer Kyle finally has Jason, his longtime heartthrob, as a boyfriend, and he seriously considers giving up Princeton so he can stay with Jason. Basketball star Jason comes out to the school, endangering the athletic scholarship he cannot afford to lose. Nelson, already worried he might be HIV positive, thinks he can solve his problems by dating Jeremy, who *is* positive. When Nelson tests negative, he *still* wants to throw himself at Jeremy. Although the story focuses equally on the three protagonists, Nelson's reckless behavior dominates, preoccupying his best friend, Kyle. Even Jeremy, who has learned from and changed his own risky behavior, is appalled; consequently he and Nelson break up as a couple, but remain friends.

HIV/AIDS is a fact of life for the young men in this novel: Safe-sex lectures at a youth group, stories of dangerous one-night stands, and taking meds are familiar territory. The sex scenes are fairly graphic. The author, a youth counselor, has a pedagogical purpose, but it is made palatable coming from characters the reader will recognize and may identify with. The photographic cover is also inviting. Like the first book, this one ends with a detailed listing of organizations geared toward teens and sexuality. [AYG]

SANCHEZ, ALEX. *Rainbow Road*. New York: Simon & Schuster, 2005. ISBN 0-689-86565-1 (hardcover)
HIV/AIDS Content Scale: Accurate
HIV/AIDS Role in Story Scale: Mentioned in passing
Literary Quality Scale: Good

This is the third book in a trilogy about three homosexual high school boys. It follows them the summer after their senior year, after Jason and Kyle have both come out. Nelson is flamboyantly out from the first book. When Jason is invited to speak at the commencement ceremony of a new high school for gay, lesbian, and transgendered students across the country, he, Kyle, and Nelson decide to take a road trip together to get there. Along the way they encounter myriad different people, problems, and opportunities. Kyle and Jason worry about Jason's lack of plan for a speech, and they also worry about Nelson, who is flighty and impulsive. Nelson worries about not having a boyfriend. The friendship dynamic changes over the course of the trip, but by the end they all realize how much they mean to each other.

The HIV content in this book is almost nonexistent, limited only to a boy featured in earlier books in the trilogy, Jeremy. The potential of becoming infected from random encounters with people whose HIV status is unknown is touched on briefly (and is notable in its gentle caution to young people), but the treatment of HIV as a topic ends there. [DC]

SAPPHIRE. *Push*. New York: Vintage Contemporaries, 1996. ISBN 0-679-44626-5 (hardcover)
HIV/AIDS Content Scale: Accurate
HIV/AIDS Role in Story Scale: Central to plot
Literary Quality Scale: Excellent

Precious Jones is sixteen and pregnant with her second child. She comes from a mind-shatteringly abusive background (both of her children are by her own father, and that is only one form of the abuse to which Precious is subjected) and as a result believes herself to be ugly and unintelligent. However, one of her teachers recognizes her potential and recommends her to an alternative school where she can learn the skills she is missing and complete the GED for graduation from high school. Her teacher there, Ms. Rain, provides a steady and loving influence in Precious's life, helping her not only with reading and writing, but also finding her shelter when baby Abdul is born and the two have no home. When Precious learns she has acquired HIV, Ms. Rain and her classmates help her push through and find hope again and a reason to live. Throughout, Precious's voice is distinct, authentic, and exquisite.

Precious was infected with HIV by her father. While the horror of this is difficult to take in an already horrifying novel, it sings with authenticity. Precious is fearful, enraged, and hopeful, and every bit of it rings true. What she knows about AIDS is impressive and skillfully delivered. The sticking point here is that her son, Abdul, ends up uninfected, although she bore him while infected and breastfed him for two years. While you cannot help but rejoice with Precious when she finds out he is perfectly healthy, this is an unusual outcome that many other similarly affected children will not share. [DC]

SCHEIDERER, ALIDA. *Of Cause and Consequence.* Scotts Valley, CA: CreateSpace, 2008. ISBN 1-438-29609-8 (paperback)
HIV/AIDS Content Scale: Accurate
HIV/AIDS Role in Story Scale: Mentioned in passing
Literary Quality Scale: Poor

It's not bad enough that Jayne Plaine feels out of it socially, she also has to deal with her nemesis Sarah Jacobson who is beautiful, rich, athletic, and mean. Sarah's favorite pastime is to make Jayne feel unpopular and freakish. More than anything, Jayne wants to know what it feels like to be the winner, and she cooks up scheme after (failed) scheme toward that end. The stakes gradually get higher and the damage more severe, but finally Jayne gets to see Sarah's excesses—unprotected sex and alcohol—start to catch up with her.

Meanwhile, the superficial friendships and trivial one-upsmanship at the center of these girls' lives are punctuated by stories of sick children and people with real problems who need help. HIV/AIDS only comes up when an HIV-positive teen speaks at an award ceremony for an organization to which both Jayne and Sarah belong. The young woman shares her regrets that she used drugs and had unprotected sex and details the price her child is paying for her bad choices. And then Jayne and Sarah have at each other once again. [MG]

SHEPHERD, PAMELA. *Zach at Risk.* New York: Alice Street Editions/Haworth Press, 2004. ISBN 1-56023-466-0 (paperback)
HIV/AIDS Content Scale: Accurate
HIV/AIDS Role in Story Scale: Central to plot
Literary Quality Scale: Passable

Zach, a young biracial Seattle teen, has an unconventional family: his mother Patrice, her female lover Dagg, and their gay friend and neighbor Josiah. Zach's mother has checked herself into a detox unit as a way of escaping from daily life, leaving Dagg and Josiah to look after Zach. But they have problems of their own: Dagg fears that Patrice has left for good, and Josiah is diagnosed with HIV. Zach starts working part-time at a comic book store and is sexually abused by Mr. Shelby, the blind owner. Raul, an older street-savvy boy who hustles for a living, befriends Zach, and together they take revenge on Mr. Shelby by trashing his store. Patrice returns. The book ends on a hopeful note, with some consolation through art and memory: Zach and Patrice drive to Washington, D.C., to deliver a panel Zach has designed, in honor of Josiah, for the AIDS quilt.

Stylistically, the book is uneven. Each chapter is headed with the name of a main character, but since all the narration is third person, the reason for this is unclear; however, it is refreshing to read a novel where lesbian parents are the norm. (Alice Street Editions is a lesbian press.) Josiah's illness is described accurately but in more graphic terms than in many of the novels; there is a horrific scene in which his legs are infested with maggots. What the novel does well is provide a social context for AIDS awareness: Josiah is one of many. [AYG]

SIMOEN, JAN. *What about Anna?* Translated from Dutch by John Nieuwenhuizen. New York: Walker & Company, 2002. [First published as *En met Anna?* in the Netherlands by Em Querido's Uitgeverij B.V. in 1999. First English-language edition published in Australia by Allen & Unwin in 2001.] ISBN 0-8027-8808-4 (hardcover)

HIV/AIDS Content Scale: Accurate
HIV/AIDS Role in Story Scale: A subplot
Literary Quality Scale: Excellent

Sixteen-year-old Anna has lost both of her brothers, Jonas to AIDS when she was eleven and Michael to a landmine two years later. The uncertainty surrounding Michael's death serves to divide what remains of Anna's family, leaving them each to cope separately and alone. Anna copes by refusing all reminders of Michael, but when a beloved friend of the family, Hugo, contacts her despite her plea to leave them all alone, she sets off once more on a quest to find a brother she had convinced herself was gone. While Anna doesn't end up connecting with Michael, she does locate Michael's old girlfriend. It is confirmed that Michael is, in fact, still alive, and he has a small son who serves as a catalyst for the family's healing process.

Jonas begins the story, after his death from AIDS. We are given no indication as to how he acquired HIV, but the portrayal of HIV is so authentic that the lack barely registers. It seems, rather, to underscore that AIDS can happen to anyone, even a best beloved sibling and friend. The people with AIDS in this novel conduct themselves with dignity, and they are treated gently and respectfully, even lovingly. However, the real triumph, the true mastery of this novel, is that it is not a novel about AIDS at all and yet the issue is covered completely, authentically, and elegantly, without taking focus away from the central plot. [DC]

STRASSER, TODD. *Can't Get There from Here.* New York: Simon & Schuster, 2004. ISBN 0-689-84169-8 (hardcover)
HIV/AIDS Content Scale: Accurate
HIV/AIDS Role in Story Scale: Mentioned in passing
Literary Quality Scale: Very good

Join life on the streets during winter in New York City. Hang out in front of the Good Life Deli with your friends Maybe, Maggot, Rainbow, 2Moro, Country Club, Tears, and OG, disposable children on their own making do with what they can find, steal, or trade for. Prostitution and drugs are a given, as is the reality that these young people will not survive a year if help is not found; however, the kind of help they have received from adults so far in their lives makes them wary of any offer of assistance on the part of authorities. One by one, they disappear, victims of violence, illness, and starvation. It is the rare child that finds his or her way home again or to any semblance of a life that might really sustain them.

HIV/AIDS is just another side deal resulting from child abuse. Meds are available from social services if street kids are savvy enough to know how to get them. It is life on the street that is deadly. [MG]

STRATTON, ALLAN. *Chanda's Secrets.* New York: Annick Press, 2004. [Canadian editorial office in Toronto.] ISBN 1-55037-835-X (hardcover)
HIV/AIDS Content Scale: Accurate
HIV/AIDS Role in Story Scale: Central to plot
Literary Quality Scale: Excellent

Against the backdrop of a fictitious Sub-Saharan African country, the threat of social isolation keeps the ill and their families from naming the killer that has them in its grip. Fear of HIV/AIDS prevents many from receiving medical and social services as well as from experiencing the love and support they need from family and friends. Sixteen-year-old Chanda is among the many who must face the choice of living in silence, being shunned, or turning away from people she loves. This is the story of Chanda's awakening to the truth of the AIDS pandemic and what happens when she decides not to keep the secret any longer.

This book presents a rare combination of powerful storytelling with accurate facts about HIV/AIDS in a plot that demonstrates the impact of HIV/AIDS on the lives of young people in Sub-Saharan Africa. The story presents HIV/AIDS as an illness that affects people of all ages, but particularly as an illness that is relevant to the young. While North American readers may not make the leap to understanding that the threat of HIV/AIDS is real for them, too, the narrative provides readers with much to think and talk about, whether this book is part of recreational or assigned reading. [MG]

STRATTON, ALLAN. *Chanda's Wars.* New York: HarperTeen, 2008. [Canadian editorial office in Toronto.] ISBN 978-0-06-087262-5 (hardcover)
HIV/AIDS Content Scale: Accurate
HIV/AIDS Role in Story Scale: Mentioned in passing
Literary Quality Scale: Good

Chanda has created a life for herself, her best friend Esther, and her younger siblings Soly and Iris in the wake of her mother's death and the estrangement from the rest of her mother's family. When Chanda's grandmother calls begging her to visit so the aging grandparents can bless the children, Chanda is conflicted. With the encouragement of those around her, however, she decides to make the journey and reconcile with the family. While they are staying with the family, Soly befriends another little boy, Pako, who recently lost his father. When Chanda discovers that the family's actual purpose in summoning her was to betroth her to the insufferable Nelson, she balks. In the meantime, civil war is breaking out across the country, and it is discovered that the ringleader is kidnapping children and forcing them to be soldiers in his army. When Pako, Soly, and Iris are kidnapped, Nelson and Chanda put aside their differences to find the children.

There is very little AIDS content in this novel, but clues interspersed throughout the text hint at the enormity of the problem. Because HIV is so stigmatized in Sub-Saharan Africa, people do not admit to having the disease, but Chanda has learned to recognize the signs. The information provided about the disease is accurate and delivered in small observations of subtle signs and symptoms that Chanda relates. [DC]

UYEMOTO, HOLLY. *Rebel without a Clue*. New York: Crown Publishers, 1989. ISBN 0-517-57170-6 (hardcover)
HIV/AIDS Content Scale: Accurate
HIV/AIDS Role in Story Scale: Central to plot
Literary Quality Scale: Passable

Christian and Thomas have been best friends for as long as they have known each other. Thomas, a talented model and actor, spends a great deal of time away from his hometown, cultivating his fame and his image. During the summer before Christian starts college, however, Thomas comes home to inform his family and Christian that he has AIDS. These are young men born to privilege, plagued with existential ennui and a superficial sophistication that is masking the fact that they are self-destructing. Unfortunately, the ennui extends to the writing itself, resulting in characters that are flat and unsympathetic and situations that never resolve themselves.

Thomas is afraid of becoming ugly as a result of the progression of AIDS. While AIDS-related weight loss feeds his vanity, he works to hide the Kaposi's sarcoma spreading over his body. Christian is morbidly afraid of contracting the disease from Thomas, with whom he does not have a sexual relationship, yet he is not at all afraid of getting it from his openly promiscuous girlfriend, who has been sexually involved with a drug dealer. The fact that Thomas has unprotected sex as a matter of course at drunken parties merits only one brief, slightly indignant comment from Christian and then is dropped. The overall message is that life is boring, so why bother protecting yourself or anybody else. Even the blatant hostility with which Thomas's stepfather addresses him after learning he has AIDS is met with barely more than an indifferent shrug. [DC]

VAN DIJK, LUTZ. *Stronger Than the Storm*. Translated from German by Karin Chubb. Cape Town: Maskew Miller Longman Pty., Ltd., 2000. [Originally published as *Township-Blues* by Elefanten Press Verlag GmbH in 2000.] ISBN 0-636-04476-9 (paperback)

HIV/AIDS Content Scale: Accurate
HIV/AIDS Role in Story Scale: Central to plot
Literary Quality Scale: Very good

Fourteen-year-old Thina (short for Thinasonke, which means "all of us together" in the Xhosa language) gets a rough start in life. She is born while her mother is in prison for refusing to turn in her politically active son, Mangaliso, to the South African authorities, who find and torture him anyway. South Africa is still under apartheid rule; however, Thina and her neighbor, Thabang, have a "friendship like the rope and the bucket. Both are necessary to get fresh milk from our cows" (p. 106). They struggle with daily life in the township of Guguletu but find strength in their romantic friendship. Both families have had their share of sorrow and hardship. Thina's traumatized older brother Mangaliso no longer speaks. Thabang's mother is ill with a mysterious illness finally diagnosed as AIDS. Thina expects that her relationship with Thabang will suffer when she is raped and subsequently contracts HIV, but it ends up being Thina's mother, not Thabang, who rejects her. However, there is hope that she will relent, and in the meantime Thina's Granny gives her blessing to Thina and Thabang for a future together.

As with other novels set in Sub-Saharan Africa, HIV/AIDS is ubiquitous and engenders many superstitions. For example, AIDS is described as punishment for promiscuity; may be cured through sex with a virgin (the idea Thina's rapist had, drunkenly, in mind); and can be passed from one family member to another. A sympathetic teacher, Miss Delphine, balances such superstitious responses by teaching her students the facts and facilitating Thina's medical care. A school play is also an effective community teaching tool. [AYG]

VELÁSQUEZ, GLORIA. *Tommy Stands Alone*. Houston, TX: Piñata Books/Arte Público Press, 1995. ISBN 1-55885-146-1 (hardcover)

HIV/AIDS Content Scale: Accurate
HIV/AIDS Role in Story Scale: A subplot
Literary Quality Scale: Poor

Tommy, a teen Latino boy, is struggling with his sexual identity among a group of high school students who have proven themselves at least mildly homophobic. His halfhearted suicide attempt convinces his friend Maya that he needs help, so she connects him with a friend of the family who is a practicing counselor. Ms. Martinez, the counselor, encourages Tommy to talk about his feelings so that he can work through them. When Tommy comes out to his mother, there is a period of deep turmoil; his mother wants him to get cured of it, and his father wants him out of the house. With the support of Maya and Ms. Martinez, however, Tommy is able to come to an understanding with his parents and grows more comfortable in his identity as a homosexual boy.

HIV does not play a role in Tommy's life, beyond the fear of pejorative homophobic AIDS-related taunts from his friends and peers. His counselor, Ms. Martinez, however, seems immersed at times in AIDS awareness, musing about the need to inform teens about safe practices, visiting the Memorial Quilt, and thinking about the people she has known or known of who had or have AIDS. There is, in fact, little discussion of the causes of HIV infection, and although Ms. Martinez's brother-in-law, Bryan, has AIDS, his partner is not infected with the virus, even though they have been together for more than five years. It seems perhaps that touching briefly on the challenges of having a partner with a different HIV status would have been appropriate, but this issue is not addressed. Although there are shortcomings in the information and the way the information present is portrayed, the overall impression is one of compassion for people with AIDS, and the impulse is to educate youth so that the cycle of infection can be halted. [DC]

WATERHOUSE, LYNDA. *Soul Love.* London: Piccadilly Press, 2004. ISBN 185340-860-3 (paperback)
HIV/AIDS Content Scale: Accurate
HIV/AIDS Role in Story Scale: A subplot
Literary Quality Scale: Very good

Jenna, in disgrace for allegedly stealing her teacher's purse, has been packed off to stay with her Aunt Sarah in the country while her mother and younger brother Marcus plan to go on holiday. Prepared to be bored all summer, Jenna discovers that the village is in fact full of intrigue. Sarah's personal and business partner Kai, a pompous poet, has left her and impregnated his new and much younger girlfriend, Emma, whose baby is due. Sarah is devastated, and Jenna ends up taking care of Sarah's bookshop as well as Sarah. Jenna is intrigued by Gabe, a young man she notices sunbathing. Gabe, the son of local landowner Lord Netherby, goes to college in London and is spending the summer in the village. Jenna ends up befriending Gabe's eccentric little sister, Aurora, and falls in love with Gabe, but in the background Gabe's friend Cleo, a waitress at the café, is always lurking.

Jenna learns that Cleo is not competition in the conventional sense. Gabe's and Cleo's mothers, now both dead, had met and become friends as patients in an AIDS hospice. Gabe and Cleo, also both HIV positive, put their particular bond above romantic relationships. Although they have a support group in London (in the village their status is still secret), they rely intensely on one another. When Cleo falls ill, Gabe chooses to go to Italy to help her recuperate rather than stay with Jenna, although it is clear that he and Jenna care for one another. In this novel, HIV/AIDS is intertwined with integrity, duty, and love. [AYG]

WIELER, DIANA. *Ran Van: Magic Nation*. Buffalo, NY: Groundwood Books/Douglas and McIntyre, 1997. [Canadian editorial office in Toronto.] ISBN 0-88899-317-X (hardcover)
HIV/AIDS Content Scale: Accurate
HIV/AIDS Role in Story Scale: A subplot
Literary Quality Scale: Excellent

In this conclusion to the Ran Van trilogy, eighteen-year-old Rhan trains for a job as a television camera operator at a highly regarded school of technology. While he still has some special abilities, this phase of life is more concerned with school life and budding romance, until he stumbles across his old adversary, Lee the Iceman. Lee asks Rhan to help him uncover a plot to kill Jim Rusk, who is channeling money to several white supremacist organizations.

Rhan later learns that Lee is HIV positive, due to exposure "in all the categories" (p. 188) and that Jim Rusk is Lee's lover; however, there is little elaboration about what it means to be HIV positive. Lee has accepted that his life span will be shortened and does not believe that he will see a cure. The main concern for transmission in this story is through exposure to infected blood resulting from physical violence. Although Rhan finds Lee's connection to these racist organizations abhorrent, the compassion and help that Rhan offers Lee are quite moving. Lee and Rhan, it turns out, are not immortal. Lee dies, not from AIDS, but in a heroic effort to save Jim Rusk, who in his turn outs the organizations that had been funding racist groups on camera for Rhan. [MG]

WOMACK, JACK. *Random Acts of Senseless Violence*. New York: Atlantic Monthly Press, 1994. [First published in Great Britain by HarperCollins in 1993.] ISBN 0-87113-577-9 (paperback)

HIV/AIDS Content Scale: Accurate
HIV/AIDS Role in Story Scale: Mentioned in passing
Literary Quality Scale: Very good

In this apocalyptic novel, twelve-year-old Lola's family falls into desperate economic circumstances, forcing them to move from their posh apartment in downtown Manhattan to a filthy flat in the ghetto. The degeneration in the world around her—marked by riots, martial law, and rampant tuberculosis and drug use—is mirrored in Lola's own degeneration and that of her family. Lola's parents are faced with imminent economic disaster. Her mother copes by living in a constant drugged stupor, and her father is repeatedly abused by his boss, until Lola finds him dead of a heart attack. Her younger sister, with whom she was once quite close, turns hostile and taciturn, eventually leaving to live with the children's aunt in California, a move that would solidify her physical and mental withdrawal from the family. Lola learns from her new friends how to live on the streets. The novel culminates in a scene of violence that marks Lola's rite of passage into the most notorious of street gangs, the Dcons.

HIV is just a small part of the hopeless tapestry constructed in this novel. Those who are infected with AIDS are homeless and begging for money. HIV is mentioned only in passing, for instance, the homeless vet who says he was in Vietnam and now has AIDS. Many of the young women in this novel prostitute themselves without any concern of infection. In fact, the use of protection may be considered superfluous, in this place where death is most likely to come quickly and violently. [DC]

YOUNG, ALIDA E. *I Never Got to Say Good-Bye.* Worthington, OH: Willowisp Press, 1988. ISBN 0-87406-359-0 (paperback)
HIV/AIDS Content Scale: Accurate
HIV/AIDS Role in Story Scale: Central to plot
Literary Quality Scale: Passable

Mark, who is more like a brother than an uncle to Traci, contracted HIV from a blood transfusion he received after a horrible automobile accident that killed his parents. Rather than face the inevitable questions and potential stigma at school, Mark quits college and moves back in with Traci and her parents. Like Mark, Traci's parents are reluctant to deal with the potential fallout that Mark's diagnosis may evoke in the community. While they offer financial support, they do their best to keep Mark's diagnosis a secret and distance themselves from him. Inevitably, word gets out, and Mark suffers a series of consequences that grow in intensity from being denied an apartment to the destruction of his personal property. A secondary character, Danny, who has AIDS due to a history of drug use, suffers much of his illness in isolation and dies alone. While not everyone in this community is without compassion for those who are HIV positive or have AIDS, they are in the minority and rarely speak up. Hostility and fear rule the day until Traci and her parents find it within themselves to stand up for Mark in a public forum and thereby win some of their own dignity back.

The strength of this story is in its exploration of how both the fear of stigma and stigma itself work to limit the lives and possibilities for people with HIV/AIDS as well as the potential of social support and education as ways for individuals to find the strength to move beyond living in fear. [MG]

ZALBEN, JANE BRESKIN. *Unfinished Dreams.* New York: Simon & Schuster Books for Young Readers, 1996. ISBN 0-689-80033-9 (hardcover)

HIV/AIDS Content Scale: Accurate

HIV/AIDS Role in Story Scale: Central to plot

Literary Quality Scale: Good

Sixth grader Jason Glass dreams of becoming a great violinist one day. His principal, Mr. Carr, has encouraged him in this and other endeavors ever since Jason started school. Jason is therefore devastated when Mr. Carr is diagnosed, not with the flu, as the school at first intimates, but with the HIV virus, and later AIDS. The book is marred by the depiction of Mr. Carr as perfect. This may be due to the author's son actually having had such an inspiring teacher; perhaps she was simply too close to her material. It is otherwise a sensitive look at how one boy, helped by his extended Jewish family, deals with various losses, including the gradual death of an important figure in his life.

Mr. Carr's HIV-positive status raises a number of issues at the school. Some parents and students blame him for having brought the illness on himself, through gay sex. One mother is particularly vicious, recommending that the school board not extend his health benefits further because he likely would not live much longer. These social ramifications of HIV/AIDS ring true, as does the description of the physical changes in Mr. Carr as his disease progresses. [AYG]

Appendix A

Young Adult Novels with HIV/AIDS Content Publication by Year

1986

Kerr, M. E. *Night Kites*. New York: HarperTrophy, 1986. ISBN 0-06-447035-0 (paperback)

1987

Miklowitz, Gloria D. *Good-Bye Tomorrow*. New York: Delacorte Press, 1987. ISBN 0-385-29562-6 (hardcover)

1988

Hoffman, Alice. *At Risk*. New York: Putnam, 1988. ISBN 0-399-13367-4 (hardcover)

Koertge, Ron. *The Arizona Kid*. Boston: Little, Brown, 1988. [Different editions have slightly different texts.] ISBN 0-7636-2542-6 (hardcover)

Young, Alida E. *I Never Got to Say Good-Bye*. Worthington, OH: Willowisp Press, 1988. ISBN 0-87406-359-0 (paperback)

1989

Hermes, Patricia. *Be Still My Heart*. New York: G. P. Putnam's Sons, 1989. ISBN 0-671-70645-4 (paperback)

Uyemoto, Holly. *Rebel without a Clue*. New York: Crown Publishers, 1989. ISBN 0-517-57170-6 (hardcover)

1990

Cohen, Miriam. *Laura Leonora's First Amendment*. New York: Lodestar Books/Dutton, 1990. ISBN 0-525-67317-2 (hardcover)

Levy, Marilyn. *Rumors and Whispers*. New York: Fawcett Juniper/Ballantine Books, 1990. ISBN 0-449-70327-4 (paperback)

1991

Gleitzman, Morris. *Two Weeks with the Queen*. New York: Putnam, 1991. [First published in Australia by Penguin Books Australia, Ltd. in 1989.] ISBN 0-141-31455-9 (paperback)

Humphreys, Martha. *Until Whatever*. New York: Clarion Books, 1991. ISBN 0-395-58022-6 (hardcover)

1992

Arrick, Fran. *What You Don't Know Can Kill You*. New York: Bantam Books, 1992. ISBN 0-440-21894-2 (paperback)

Durant, Penny Raife. *When Heroes Die*. New York: Atheneum, 1992. ISBN 0-689-31764-6 (hardcover)

Hunt, Angela Elwell. *A Dream to Cherish*. Cassie Perkins Series, No. 4. Lincoln, NE: Authors Guild Backinprint.com Edition/iUniverse.com, 1992. [First published by Tyndale House Publishers.] ISBN 0-595-08995-X (paperback)

McDaniel, Lurlene. *Sixteen and Dying*. (One Last Wish). New York: Bantam, 1992. ISBN 0-553-29932-8 (paperback)

St. John, Charlotte. *Red Hair Three*. New York: Fawcett Juniper, 1992. ISBN 0-449-70406-8 (paperback)

1993

Baer, Judy. *The Discovery*. Cedar River Daydreams, No. 20. Minneapolis: Bethany House, 1993. ISBN 1-55661-330-X (paperback)

Bess, Clayton. *The Mayday Rampage*. Sacramento, CA: Lookout Press, 1993. ISBN 1-882405-00-5 (hardcover)

Kaye, Marilyn. *Real Heroes*. New York: Harcourt Brace Jovanovich, 1993. ISBN 0-15-200563-3 (hardcover)

Lennon, Tom. *When Love Comes to Town*. Dublin: O'Brien Press, 1993. ISBN 0-86278-361-5 (paperback)

McDaniel, Lurlene. *Baby Alicia Is Dying*. New York: Bantam, 1993. ISBN 0-553-29605-1 (paperback)

Roper, Gayle. *The Case of the Missing Melody*. East Edge Mysteries, No. 4. Elgin, IL: Chariot Books/David C. Cook Publishing Co., 1993. ISBN 1-55513-702-4 (paperback)

1994

Benning, Elizabeth. [Pseudonym for Alida E. Young.] *Losing David*. New York: Harper Paperbacks, 1994. ISBN 0-06-106147-6 (paperback)

Davis, Deborah. *My Brother Has AIDS*. New York: Jean Karl/Atheneum, 1994. ISBN 0-689-31922-3 (hardcover)

Johnson, Scott. *Overnight Sensation*. New York: Atheneum, 1994. ISBN 0-689-31831-6 (hardcover)

McClain, Ellen Jaffe. *No Big Deal*. New York: Lodestar Books, 1994. ISBN 0-525-67483-7 (paperback)

Nelson, Theresa. *Earthshine*. New York: Orchard Books, 1994. ISBN 0-531-06867-6 (hardcover)

Paulsen, Gary. *The Car*. Orlando, FL: Harcourt Brace & Company, 1994. ISBN 0-15-292878-2 (hardcover)

Pike, Christopher. *The Last Vampire*. New York: Archway Paperbacks, 1994. ISBN 0-671-87264-8 (paperback)

Pike, Christopher. *The Midnight Club*. New York: Archway Paperbacks, 1994. ISBN 0-671-87263-X (paperback)

Porte, Barbara Ann. *Something Terrible Happened*. New York: Orchard Books, 1994. ISBN 0-531-06869-2 (hardcover)

Roper, Gayle. *The Mystery of the Poison Pen*. East Edge Mysteries, No. 5. Elgin, IL: Chariot Books/David C. Cook Publishing Co., 1994. ISBN 0-7814-1507-1 (paperback)

Womack, Jack. *Random Acts of Senseless Violence*. New York: Atlantic Monthly Press, 1994. [First published in Great Britain by HarperCollins in 1993.] ISBN 0-87113-577-9 (paperback)

1995

Bantle, Lee F. *Diving for the Moon*. New York: Macmillan Books for Young Readers, 1995. ISBN 0-689-80004-5 (hardcover)

Fox, Paula. *The Eagle Kite*. New York: Orchard Books, 1995. ISBN 0-531-06892-7 (hardcover)

Peck, Richard. *The Last Safe Place on Earth*. New York: Delacorte Press, 1995. ISBN 0-385-32052-3 (hardcover)

Pinsker, Judith. *Robin's Diary*. Radnor, PA: ABC Daytime Press/ Chilton Book Company, 1995. [Based on the story by Claire Labine.] ISBN 0-8019-8775-X (paperback)

Velásquez, Gloria. *Tommy Stands Alone*. Houston, TX: Piñata Books/Arte Público Press, 1995. ISBN 1-55885-146-1 (hardcover)

1996

Cooper, Melrose. *Life Magic*. New York: Henry Holt and Company, 1996. ISBN 0-8050-4114-1 (hardcover)

Hobbs, Valerie. *Get It While It's Hot. Or Not*. New York: Richard Jackson/Orchard, 1996. ISBN 0-531-09540-1 (hardcover)

Maguire, Gregory. *Oasis*. New York: Clarion Books, 1996. ISBN 0-395-67019-5 (hardcover)

Sapphire. *Push*. New York: Vintage Contemporaries, 1996. ISBN 0-679-44626-5 (hardcover)

Zalben, Jane Breskin. *Unfinished Dreams*. New York: Simon & Schuster Books for Young Readers, 1996. ISBN 0-689-80033-9 (hardcover)

1997

Wieler, Diana. *Ran Van: Magic Nation*. Buffalo, NY: Groundwood Books/Douglas and McIntyre, 1997. [Canadian editorial office in Toronto.] ISBN 0-88899-317-X (hardcover)

1998

Block, Francesca Lia. *I Was a Teenage Fairy*. New York: Joanna Cotler Books/HarperCollins, 1998. ISBN 0-06-027747-5 (hardcover)

Hernández, Irene Beltrán. *Woman Soldier/La Soldadera*. Waco, TX: Blue Rose Books, 1998. ISBN 0-9676833-0-0 (paperback)

Peck, Richard. *Strays Like Us*. New York: Puffin Books, 1998. ISBN 0-8037-2291-5 (hardcover)

1999

Bennett, Cherie, and Gottesfeld, Jeff. *University Hospital: Condition Critical*. Book Two. New York: Berkley Jam Books, 1999. ISBN 0-425-17256-2 (paperback)

Huser, Glen. *Touch of the Clown*. Buffalo, NY: Groundwood, 1999. [Canadian editorial office in Toronto.] ISBN 0-88899-343-9 (hardcover)

Mitchell, Nancy. *Raging Skies*. Changing Earth Trilogy, Book Two. Fremont, CA: Lightstream Publications, 1999. ISBN 1-892713-01-2 (paperback)

Rivers, Karen. *Dream Water*. Custer, WA: Orca Book Publishers, 1999. [Canadian editorial office in Victoria, BC.] ISBN 1-55143-160-2 (hardcover)

2000

Bennett, Cherie, and Gottesfeld, Jeff. *University Hospital: Crisis Point*. Book Three. New York: Berkley Jam Books, 2000. ISBN 0-425-17338-0 (paperback)

Bennett, Cherie, and Gottesfeld, Jeff. *University Hospital: Heart Trauma*. Book Four. New York: Berkley Jam Books, 2000. ISBN: 0-425-17404-2 (paperback)

Eliot, Eve. *Insatiable: The Compelling Story of Four Teens, Food, and Its Power*. Deerfield Beach, FL: Health Communications, 2001. ISBN 1-55874-818-0 (paperback)

Field, Barbara. *The Deeper, the Bluer*. Lincoln, NE: iUniverse .com, 2000. ISBN 0-595-13378-9 (paperback)

Van Dijk, Lutz. *Stronger Than the Storm*. Translated from German by Karin Chubb. Cape Town: Maskew Miller Longman Pty., Ltd., 2000. [Originally published as *Township-Blues* by Elefanten Press Verlag GmbH in 2000.] ISBN 0-636-04476-9 (paperback)

2001

Dow, Unity. *Far and Beyon'*. San Francisco: Aunt Lute Books, 2001. [First published by Longman, Botswana Pty., Ltd. in December 2000. This edition published in North Melbourne, Australia, in conjunction with Spinifex Press Pty., Ltd., in 2001.] ISBN 1-879960-64-8 (paperback)

Hansen, Joyce. *One True Friend*. New York: Clarion, 2001. ISBN 0-395-84983-7 (hardcover)

Nolan, Han. *Born Blue*. New York: Harcourt, 2001. ISBN 0-15-201916-2 (hardcover)

Sanchez, Alex. *Rainbow Boys*. New York: Simon & Schuster, 2001. ISBN 0-689-85770-5 (paperback)

2002

Bennett, Cherie, and Gottesfeld, Jeff. *University Hospital: Prognosis: Heartbreak*. Book Five. New York: Berkley Jam Books, 2002. ISBN 0-425-18147-2 (paperback)

Goodman, Alison. *Singing the Dogstar Blues*. New York: Viking, 2002. [First published by Voyager, an imprint of HarperCollins Publishers Australia, in 1998.] ISBN 0-670-03610-2 (hardcover)

Mankell, Henning. *Playing with Fire*. Translated from Swedish by Anna Paterson. Crows Nest, NSW, Australia: Allen & Unwin, 2002. [First published as *Eldens Gåta* by Rabén & Sjögren Bokförlag in Sweden in 2001.] ISBN 1-86508-714-9 (paperback)

Moore, Stephanie Perry. *Laurel Shadrach Series 1: Purity Reigns*. Chicago: Moody Press, 2002. ISBN 0-8024-4035-5 (paperback)

Moore, Stephanie Perry. *Laurel Shadrach Series 2: Totally Free*. Chicago: Moody Press, 2002. ISBN 0-8024-4036-3 (paperback)

Plum-Ucci, Carol. *What Happened to Lani Garver*. Orlando, FL: Harcourt, 2002. ISBN 0-15-216813-3 (hardcover)

Simoen, Jan. *What about Anna?* Translated from Dutch by John Nieuwenhuizen. New York: Walker & Company, 2002. [First published as *En met Anna?* in the Netherlands by Em Querido's Uitgeverij B.V. in 1999. First English-language edition published in Australia by Allen & Unwin in 2001.] ISBN 0-8027-8808-4 (hardcover)

2003

Brockton, Quinn. *Never Tear Us Apart*. A "Queer as Folk" Novel. New York: Pocket Books/Simon & Schuster, 2003. ISBN 0-7434-7613-1 (paperback)

Harley, Rex. *Now That I've Found You*. Llandysul, Ceredigion, Wales: Pont Books/Gomer Press, 2003. ISBN 1-85902-107-7 (paperback)

Moore, Stephanie Perry. *Laurel Shadrach Series 3: Equally Yoked*. Chicago: Moody Publishers, 2003. ISBN 0-8024-4037-1 (paperback)

Moore, Stephanie Perry. *Laurel Shadrach Series 4: Absolutely Worthy*. Chicago: Moody Publishers, 2003. ISBN 0-8024-4038-X (paperback)

Sanchez, Alex. *Rainbow High*. New York: Simon Pulse, 2003. ISBN 0-689-85477-3 (hardcover)

2004

Ellis, Deborah. *The Heaven Shop*. Allston, MA: Fitzhenry & Whiteside, 2004. [Canadian editorial office in Markham, Ontario.] ISBN 1-55041-908-0 (hardcover)

Hood, Rob N. *Beyond the Wind*. Binghamton, NY: Southern Tier Editions/Harrington Park Press/Haworth Press, 2004. ISBN-10 1-56023-482-2; ISBN-13 978-1-56023-482-1 (paperback)

Minchin, Adele. *The Beat Goes On*. New York: Simon & Schuster, 2004. [First published in Great Britain by Livewire Books, the Women's Press Limited, in 2001.] ISBN 0-689-86611-9 (hardcover)

Moore, Stephanie Perry. *Laurel Shadrach Series 5: Finally Sure*. Chicago: Moody Publishers, 2004. ISBN 0-8024-4039-8 (paperback)

Shepherd, Pamela. *Zach at Risk*. New York: Alice Street Editions/Haworth Press, 2004. ISBN 1-56023-466-0 (paperback)

Strasser, Todd. *Can't Get There from Here*. New York: Simon & Schuster, 2004. ISBN 0-689-84169-8 (hardcover)

Stratton, Allan. *Chanda's Secrets*. New York: Annick Press, 2004. [Canadian editorial office in Toronto.] ISBN 1-55037-835-X (hardcover)

Waterhouse, Lynda. *Soul Love*. London: Piccadilly Press, 2004. ISBN 185340-860-3 (paperback)

2005

Babcock, Joe. *The Tragedy of Miss Geneva Flowers*. New York: Carroll & Graf Publishers, 2005. [First published by Joe Babcock in 2002.] ISBN 0-7867-1520-0 (paperback)

Chase, Barbara. *The Silent Killer*. Kingston, Jamaica: Ian Randle Publishers, 2005. [First edition published in 2000. Revised edition published in 2002.] ISBN 976-637-179-2 (paperback)

Flinn, Alex. *Fade to Black*. New York: HarperTempest, 2005. ISBN 0-06-056839-9 (hardcover)

Sanchez, Alex. *Rainbow Road*. New York: Simon & Schuster, 2005. ISBN 0-689-86565-1 (hardcover)

2006

First Born. [Pseudonym for Brian Williams.] *Delivered from Evil*. Bloomington, IN: Trafford Publishing, 2006. ISBN 1-4120-8048-7 (paperback)

Gonzales, S. Bryan. *Under the Big Sky*. Bloomington, IN: Author House, 2006. ISBN-10 1-425-96524-5; ISBN-13 978-1-4259-6524-2 (paperback)

2007

Carlson, Melody. *Notes from a Spinning Planet: Papua New Guinea*. Colorado Springs, CO: WaterBrook Press/Random House, 2007. ISBN 978-1-40000-7145-6 (paperback)

Sanchez, Alex. *The God Box*. New York: Simon & Schuster Books for Young Readers, 2007. ISBN-10 1-4169-0899-4; ISBN-13 978-1-4169-0899-9 (hardcover)

2008

Chase, Dakota. *Changing Jamie*. Round Rock, TX: Prizm Books/ Torquere Press, 2008. [Copyright 2007.] ISBN 1-60370-351-9 (paperback)

Doctorow, Cory. *Little Brother*. New York: Tor Teen, 2008. ISBN-10 0-7653-1985-3; ISBN-13 978-0-7653-1985-2 (hardcover)

Doherty, Berlie. *The Girl Who Saw Lions*. New York: Neal Porter/ Roaring Brook Press, 2008. [First published in Great Britain by Andersen Press, Ltd.] ISBN-10 1-59643-377-9; ISBN-13 978-1-59643-377-9 (hardcover)

Scheiderer, Alida. *Of Cause and Consequence*. Scotts Valley, CA: CreateSpace, 2008. ISBN 1-438-29609-8 (paperback)

Stratton, Allan. *Chanda's Wars*. New York: HarperTeen, 2008. [Canadian editorial office in Toronto.] ISBN 978-0-06-087262-5 (hardcover)

Appendix B

Young Adult Novels in Which HIV/AIDS Is Central to the Story

Arrick, Fran. *What You Don't Know Can Kill You*. New York: Bantam Books, 1992. ISBN 0-440-21894-2 (paperback)

Baer, Judy. *The Discovery*. Cedar River Daydreams, No. 20. Minneapolis: Bethany House, 1993. ISBN 1-55661-330-X (paperback)

Bantle, Lee F. *Diving for the Moon*. New York: Macmillan Books for Young Readers, 1995. ISBN 0-689-80004-5 (hardcover)

Benning, Elizabeth. [Pseudonym for Alida E. Young.] *Losing David*. New York: Harper Paperbacks, 1994. ISBN 0-06-106147-6 (paperback)

Bess, Clayton. *The Mayday Rampage*. Sacramento, CA: Lookout Press, 1993. ISBN 1-882405-00-5 (hardcover)

Carlson, Melody. *Notes from a Spinning Planet: Papua New Guinea*. Colorado Springs, CO: WaterBrook Press/Random House, 2007. ISBN 978-1-40000-7145-6 (paperback)

Chase, Barbara. *The Silent Killer*. Kingston, Jamaica: Ian Randle Publishers, 2005. [First edition published in 2000. Revised edition published in 2002.] ISBN 976-637-179-2 (paperback)

Cohen, Miriam. *Laura Leonora's First Amendment*. New York: Lodestar Books/Dutton, 1990. ISBN 0-525-67317-2 (hardcover)

Cooper, Melrose. *Life Magic*. New York: Henry Holt and Company, 1996. ISBN 0-8050-4114-1 (hardcover)

Davis, Deborah. *My Brother Has AIDS*. New York: Jean Karl/Atheneum, 1994. ISBN 0-689-31922-3 (hardcover)

Dow, Unity. *Far and Beyon'*. San Francisco: Aunt Lute Books, 2001. [First published by Longman, Botswana Pty., Ltd., in

2000. This edition published in North Melbourne, Australia, in conjunction with Spinifex Press Pty., Ltd., in 2001.] ISBN 1-879960-64-8 (paperback)

Durant, Penny Raife. *When Heroes Die*. New York: Atheneum, 1992. ISBN 0-689-31764-6 (hardcover)

Ellis, Deborah. *The Heaven Shop*. Allston, MA: Fitzhenry & Whiteside, 2004. [Canadian editorial office in Markham, Ontario.] ISBN 1-55041-908-0 (hardcover)

Flinn, Alex. *Fade to Black*. New York: HarperTempest, 2005. ISBN 0-06-056839-9 (hardcover)

Fox, Paula. *The Eagle Kite*. New York: Orchard Books, 1995. ISBN 0-531-06892-7 (hardcover)

Hoffman, Alice. *At Risk*. New York: Putnam, 1988. ISBN 0-399-13367-4 (hardcover)

Hood, Rob N. *Beyond the Wind*. Southern Tier Editions/Harrington Park Press/Haworth Press, 2004. ISBN 1-56023-482-2 (paperback)

Humphreys, Martha. *Until Whatever*. New York: Clarion Books, 1991. ISBN 0-395-58022-6 (hardcover)

Hunt, Angela Elwell. *A Dream to Cherish*. Cassie Perkins Series, No. 4. Lincoln, NE: Authors Guild Backinprint.com Edition/iUniverse.com, 1992. [First published by Tyndale House Publishers.] ISBN 0-595-08995-X (paperback)

Huser, Glen. *Touch of the Clown*. Buffalo, NY: Groundwood, 1999. [Canadian editorial office in Toronto.] ISBN 0-88899-343-9 (hardcover)

Kaye, Marilyn. *Real Heroes*. New York: Harcourt Brace Jovanovich, 1993. ISBN 0-15-200563-3 (hardcover)

Kerr, M. E. *Night Kites*. New York: HarperTrophy, 1986. ISBN 0-06-447035-0 (paperback)

Levy, Marilyn. *Rumors and Whispers*. New York: Fawcett Juniper/Ballantine Books, 1990. ISBN 0-449-70327-4 (paperback)

McDaniel, Lurlene. *Baby Alicia Is Dying*. New York: Bantam, 1993. ISBN 0-553-29605-1 (paperback)

McDaniel, Lurlene. *Sixteen and Dying*. (One Last Wish). New York: Bantam, 1992. ISBN 0-553-29932-8 (paperback)

Maguire, Gregory. *Oasis*. New York: Clarion Books, 1996. ISBN 0-395-67019-5 (hardcover)

Mankell, Henning. *Playing with Fire*. Translated from Swedish by Anna Paterson. Crows Nest, NSW, Australia: Allen

& Unwin, 2002. [First published as *Eldens Gåta* in Sweden by Rabén & Sjögren Bokförlag in 2001.] ISBN 1-86508-714-9 (paperback)

Miklowitz, Gloria D. *Good-Bye Tomorrow*. New York: Delacorte Press, 1987. ISBN 0-385-29562-6 (hardcover)

Minchin, Adele. *The Beat Goes On*. New York: Simon & Schuster, 2004. [First published in Great Britain by Livewire Books, the Women's Press Limited, in 2001.] ISBN 0-689-86611-9 (hardcover)

Nelson, Theresa. *Earthshine*. New York: Orchard Books, 1994. ISBN 0-531-06867-6 (hardcover)

Pinsker, Judith. *Robin's Diary*. Radnor, PA: ABC Daytime Press/ Chilton Book Company, 1995. [Based on the story by Claire Labine.] ISBN 0-8019-8775-X (paperback)

Roper, Gayle. *The Mystery of the Poison Pen*. East Edge Mysteries, No. 5. Elgin, IL: Chariot Books/David C. Cook Publishing Co., 1994. ISBN 0-7814-1507-1 (paperback)

St. John, Charlotte. *Red Hair Three*. New York: Fawcett Juniper, 1992. ISBN 0-449-70406-8 (paperback)

Sapphire. *Push*. New York: Vintage Contemporaries, 1996. ISBN 0-679-44626-5 (hardcover)

Shepherd, Pamela. *Zach at Risk*. New York: Alice Street Editions/Haworth Press, 2004. ISBN 1-56023-466-0 (paperback)

Stratton, Allan. *Chanda's Secrets*. New York: Annick Press, 2004. [Canadian editorial office in Toronto.] ISBN 1-55037-835-X (hardcover)

Uyemoto, Holly. *Rebel without a Clue*. New York: Crown Publishers, 1989. ISBN 0-517-57170-6 (hardcover)

Van Dijk, Lutz. *Stronger Than the Storm*. Translated from German by Karin Chubb. Cape Town: Maskew Miller Longman Pty., Ltd., 2000. [Originally published as *Township-Blues* by Elefanten Press Verlag GmbH in 2000.] ISBN 0-636-04476-9 (paperback)

Young, Alida E. *I Never Got to Say Good-Bye*. Worthington, OH: Willowisp Press, 1988. ISBN 0-87406-359-0 (paperback)

Zalben, Jane Breskin. *Unfinished Dreams*. New York: Simon & Schuster Books for Young Readers, 1996. ISBN 0-689-80033-9 (hardcover)

Appendix C

Young Adult Novels in Which HIV/AIDS Is a Subplot in the Story

Babcock, Joe. *The Tragedy of Miss Geneva Flowers*. New York: Carroll & Graf Publishers, 2005. [First published by Joe Babcock in 2002.] ISBN 0-7867-1520-0 (paperback)

Bennett, Cherie, and Gottesfeld, Jeff. *University Hospital: Crisis Point*. Book Three. New York: Berkley Jam Books, 2000. ISBN 0-425-17338-0 (paperback)

Brockton, Quinn. *Never Tear Us Apart*. A "Queer as Folk" Novel. New York: Pocket Books/Simon & Schuster, 2003. ISBN 0-7434-7613-1 (paperback)

Chase, Dakota. *Changing Jamie*. Round Rock, TX: Prizm Books/Torquere Press, 2008. [Copyright 2007.] ISBN 1-60370-351-9 (paperback)

Doherty, Berlie. *The Girl Who Saw Lions*. New York: Neal Porter/Roaring Brook Press, 2008. [First published in Great Britain by Andersen Press, Ltd.] ISBN 1-59643-377-9 (hardcover)

Field, Barbara. *The Deeper, the Bluer*. Lincoln, NE: iUniverse.com, 2000. ISBN 0-595-13378-9 (paperback)

Gleitzman, Morris. *Two Weeks with the Queen*. New York: Putnam, 1991. [First published in Australia by Penguin Books Australia, Ltd. in 1989.] ISBN 0-141-31455-9 (paperback)

Hansen, Joyce. *One True Friend*. New York: Clarion, 2001. ISBN 0-395-84983-7 (hardcover)

Harley, Rex. *Now That I've Found You*. Llandysul, Ceredigion, Wales: Pont Books/Gomer Press, 2003. ISBN 1-85902-107-7 (paperback)

Hermes, Patricia. *Be Still My Heart*. New York: G. P. Putnam's Sons, 1989. ISBN 0-671-70645-4 (paperback)

Hernández, Irene Beltrán. *Woman Soldier/La Soldadera*. Waco, TX: Blue Rose Books, 1998. ISBN 0-9676833-0-0 (paperback)

Hobbs, Valerie. *Get It While It's Hot. Or Not*. New York: Richard Jackson/Orchard, 1996. ISBN 0-531-09540-1 (hardcover)

Koertge, Ron. *The Arizona Kid*. Boston: Little, Brown, 1988. [Different editions have slightly different texts.] ISBN 0-7636-2542-6 (hardcover)

Lennon, Tom. *When Love Comes to Town*. Dublin: O'Brien Press, 1993. ISBN 0-86278-361-5 (paperback)

McClain, Ellen Jaffe. *No Big Deal*. New York: Lodestar Books, 1994. ISBN 0-525-67483-7 (paperback)

Mitchell, Nancy. *Raging Skies*. Changing Earth Trilogy, Book Two. Fremont, CA: Lightstream Publications, 1999. ISBN 1-892713-01-2 (paperback)

Moore, Stephanie Perry. *Laurel Shadrach Series 2: Totally Free*. Chicago: Moody Press, 2002. ISBN 0-8024-4036-3 (paperback)

Nolan, Han. *Born Blue*. New York: Harcourt, 2001. ISBN 0-15-201916-2 (hardcover)

Peck, Richard. *Strays Like Us*. New York: Puffin Books, 1998. ISBN 0-8037-2291-5 (hardcover)

Pike, Christopher. *The Last Vampire*. New York: Archway Paperbacks, 1994. ISBN 0-671-87264-8 (paperback)

Pike, Christopher. *The Midnight Club*. New York: Archway Paperbacks, 1994. ISBN 0-671-87263-X (paperback)

Porte, Barbara Ann. *Something Terrible Happened*. New York: Orchard Books, 1994. ISBN 0-531-06869-2 (hardcover)

Rivers, Karen. *Dream Water*. Custer, WA: Orca Book Publishers, 1999. [Canadian editorial office in Victoria, BC.] ISBN 1-55143-160-2 (hardcover)

Sanchez, Alex. *Rainbow Boys*. New York: Simon & Schuster, 2001. ISBN 0-689-85770-5 (paperback)

Sanchez, Alex. *Rainbow High*. New York: Simon Pulse, 2003. ISBN 0-689-85477-3 (hardcover)

Simoen, Jan. *What about Anna?* Translated from Dutch by John Nieuwenhuizen. New York: Walker & Company, 2002. [First published as *En met Anna?* in the Netherlands by Em Querido's Uitgeverij B.V. in 1999. First English-language edition published in Australia by Allen & Unwin in 2001.] ISBN 0-8027-8808-4 (hardcover)

Velásquez, Gloria. *Tommy Stands Alone*. Houston, TX: Piñata Books/Arte Público Press, 1995. ISBN 1-55885-146-1 (hardcover)

Waterhouse, Lynda. *Soul Love*. London: Piccadilly Press, 2004. ISBN 185340-860-3 (paperback)

Wieler, Diana. *Ran Van: Magic Nation*. Buffalo, NY: Groundwood Books/Douglas & McIntyre, 1997. [Canadian editorial office in Toronto.] ISBN 0-88899-317-X (hardcover)

Appendix D

Young Adult Novels in Which HIV/AIDS Is Mentioned in Passing

Bennett, Cherie, and Gottesfeld, Jeff. *University Hospital: Condition Critical*. Book Two. New York: Berkley Jam Books, 1999. ISBN 0-425-17256-2 (paperback)

Bennett, Cherie, and Gottesfeld, Jeff. *University Hospital: Heart Trauma*. Book Four. New York: Berkley Jam Books, 2000. ISBN 0-425-17404-2 (paperback)

Bennett, Cherie, and Gottesfeld, Jeff. *University Hospital: Prognosis: Heartbreak*. Book Five. New York: Berkley Jam Books, 2002. ISBN 0-425-18147-2 (paperback)

Block, Francesca Lia. *I Was a Teenage Fairy*. New York: Joanna Cotler Books/HarperCollins, 1998. ISBN 0-06-027747-5 (hardcover)

Doctorow, Cory. *Little Brother*. New York: Tor Teen, 2008. ISBN 0-7653-1985-3 (hardcover)

Eliot, Eve. *Insatiable: The Compelling Story of Four Teens, Food, and Its Power*. Deerfield Beach, FL: Health Communications, 2001. ISBN 1-55874-818-0 (paperback)

First Born. [Pseudonym for Brian Williams.] *Delivered from Evil*. Bloomington, IN: Trafford Publishing, 2006. ISBN 1-4120-8048-7 (paperback)

Gonzales, S. Bryan. *Under the Big Sky*. Bloomington, IN: AuthorHouse, 2006. ISBN 1-425-96524-5 (paperback)

Goodman, Alison. *Singing the Dogstar Blues*. New York: Viking, 2002. [First published by Voyager, an imprint of HarperCollins Publishers Australia, in 1998.] ISBN 0-670-03610-2 (hardcover)

Johnson, Scott. *Overnight Sensation*. New York: Atheneum, 1994. ISBN 0-689-31831-6 (hardcover)

Moore, Stephanie Perry. *Laurel Shadrach Series 1: Purity Reigns*. Chicago: Moody Press, 2002. ISBN 0-8024-4035-5 (paperback)

Moore, Stephanie Perry. *Laurel Shadrach Series 3: Equally Yoked*. Chicago: Moody Publishers, 2003. ISBN 0-8024-4037-1 (paperback)

Moore, Stephanie Perry. *Laurel Shadrach Series 4: Absolutely Worthy*. Chicago: Moody Publishers, 2003. ISBN 0-8024-4038-X (paperback)

Moore, Stephanie Perry. *Laurel Shadrach Series 5: Finally Sure*. Chicago: Moody Publishers, 2004. ISBN 0-8024-4039-8 (paperback)

Paulsen, Gary. *The Car*. Orlando, FL: Harcourt Brace & Company, 1994. ISBN 0-15-292878-2 (hardcover)

Peck, Richard. *The Last Safe Place on Earth*. New York: Delacorte Press, 1995. ISBN 0-385-32052-3 (hardcover)

Plum-Ucci, Carol. *What Happened to Lani Garver*. Orlando, FL: Harcourt, 2002. ISBN 0-15-216813-3 (hardcover)

Roper, Gayle. *The Case of the Missing Melody*. East Edge Mysteries, No. 4. Elgin, IL: Chariot Books/David C. Cook Publishing Co., 1993. ISBN 1-55513-702-4 (paperback)

Sanchez, Alex. *The God Box*. New York: Simon & Schuster Books for Young Readers, 2007. ISBN 1-4169-0899-4 (hardcover)

Sanchez, Alex. *Rainbow Road*. New York: Simon & Schuster, 2005. ISBN 0-689-86565-1 (hardcover)

Scheiderer, Alida. *Of Cause and Consequence*. Scotts Valley, CA: CreateSpace, 2008. ISBN 1-438-29609-8 (paperback)

Strasser, Todd. *Can't Get There from Here*. New York: Simon & Schuster, 2004. ISBN 0-689-84169-8 (hardcover)

Stratton, Allan. *Chanda's Wars*. New York: HarperTeen, 2008. [Canadian editorial office in Toronto.] ISBN 978-0-06-087262-5 (hardcover)

Womack, Jack. *Random Acts of Senseless Violence*. New York: Atlantic Monthly Press, 1994. [First published in Great Britain by HarperCollins in 1993.] ISBN 0-87113-577-9 (paperback)

Appendix E

Books First Published Outside the United States

Chase, Barbara. *The Silent Killer*. Kingston, Jamaica: Ian Randle Publishers, 2005. [First edition published in 2000. Revised edition published in 2002.] ISBN 976-637-179-2 (paperback)

Doherty, Berlie. *The Girl Who Saw Lions*. New York: Neal Porter/Roaring Brook Press, 2008. [First published in Great Britain by Andersen Press, Ltd.] ISBN-10 1-59643-377-9 (hardcover)

Dow, Unity. *Far and Beyon'*. San Francisco: Aunt Lute Books, 2001. [First published by Longman, Botswana Pty., Ltd. in 2000. This edition published in North Melbourne, Australia, in conjunction with Spinifex Press Pty., Ltd., in 2001.] ISBN 1-879960-64-8 (paperback)

Ellis, Deborah. *The Heaven Shop*. Allston, MA: Fitzhenry & Whiteside, 2004. [Canadian editorial office in Markham, Ontario.] ISBN 1-55041-908-0 (hardcover)

Gleitzman, Morris. *Two Weeks with the Queen*. New York: Putnam, 1991. [First published in Australia by Penguin Books Australia, Ltd. in 1989.] ISBN 0-141-31455-9 (paperback)

Goodman, Alison. *Singing the Dogstar Blues*. New York: Viking, 2002. [First published by Voyager, an imprint of HarperCollins Publishers Australia, in 1998.] ISBN 0-670-03610-2 (hardcover)

Harley, Rex. *Now That I've Found You*. Llandysul, Ceredigion, Wales: Pont Books/Gomer Press, 2003. ISBN 1-85902-107-7 (paperback)

Huser, Glen. *Touch of the Clown*. Buffalo, NY: Groundwood, 1999. [Canadian editorial office in Toronto.] ISBN 0-88899-343-9 (hardcover)

Lennon, Tom. *When Love Comes to Town*. Dublin: O'Brien Press, 1993. ISBN 0-86278-361-5 (paperback)

Mankell, Henning. *Playing with Fire*. Translated from Swedish by Anna Paterson. Crows Nest, NSW, Australia: Allen & Unwin, 2002. [First published as *Eldens Gåta* in Sweden by Rabén & Sjögren Bokförlag in 2001.] ISBN 1-86508-714-9 (paperback)

Minchin, Adele. *The Beat Goes On*. New York: Simon & Schuster, 2004. [First published in Great Britain by Livewire Books, the Women's Press Limited, in 2001.] ISBN 0-689-86611-9 (hardcover)

Rivers, Karen. *Dream Water*. Custer, WA: Orca Book Publishers, 1999. [Canadian editorial office in Victoria, BC.] ISBN 1-55143-160-2 (hardcover)

Simoen, Jan. *What about Anna?* Translated from Dutch by John Nieuwenhuizen. New York: Walker & Company, 2002. [First published as *En met Anna?* in the Netherlands by Em Querido's Uitgeverij B.V. in 1999. First English-language edition published in Australia by Allen & Unwin in 2001.] ISBN 0-8027-8808-4 (hardcover)

Stratton, Allan. *Chanda's Secrets*. New York: Annick Press, 2004. [Canadian editorial office in Toronto.] ISBN 1-55037-835-X (hardcover)

Stratton, Allan. *Chanda's Wars*. New York: HarperTeen, 2008. [Canadian editorial office in Toronto.] ISBN 978-0-06-087262-5 (hardcover)

Van Dijk, Lutz. *Stronger Than the Storm*. Translated from German by Karin Chubb. Cape Town: Maskew Miller Longman Pty., Ltd., 2000. [Originally published as *Township-Blues* by Elefanten Press Verlag GmbH in 2000.] ISBN 0-636-04476-9 (paperback)

Waterhouse, Lynda. *Soul Love*. London: Piccadilly Press, 2004. ISBN 185340-860-3 (paperback)

Wieler, Diana. *Ran Van: Magic Nation*. Buffalo, NY: Groundwood Books/Douglas & McIntyre, 1997. [Canadian editorial office in Toronto.] ISBN 0-88899-317-X (hardcover)

Womack, Jack. *Random Acts of Senseless Violence*. New York: Atlantic Monthly Press, 1994. [First published in Great Britain by HarperCollins in 1993.] ISBN 0-87113-577-9 (paperback)

Appendix F

Coding Sheets

Note: Versions of the coding sheets for Who Has HIVAIDS in These Novels, How Did HIV/AIDS Characters Get Infected, What Are the Explicit Fears of Protagonists Concerning HIV/AIDS, and What Is the Fate of HIV/AIDS Characters in These Stories originally appeared in Melissa Gross, "What Do Young Adult Novels Say about HIV/AIDS?" Library Quarterly *68, no.1 (1998): 26–28, copyright 1998 by the University of Chicago.*

WHO HAS HIV/AIDS IN THESE NOVELS?

Book Title: ______________________ Coder Name: ______________

Relationship of HIV/AIDS Character to Protagonist	*Relevant Content*	*Page(s)*
1. No direct relationship		
2. Extended family member (aunt, uncle, cousin, grandparent)		
3. Immediate family member (parent, sister, brother)		
4. Family friend		
5. Friend (strong personal attachment, not a love interest)		
6. Love interest		
7. Classmate (limited personal attachment, in same peer group)		
8. Teacher		
9. Teacher's family/friend		
10. Self		
11. Other (see identified subcategories below)		
Number male/ number female		
Age(s) of character(s) with HIV/AIDS		
Total number of characters with HIV/AIDS presented in story		

HOW DID HIV/AIDS CHARACTERS GET INFECTED?

Book Title: ______________________________ Coder Name: ________________

Cause/Names	*How Contracted*	*Pages(s)*	*Evidence of Infection*	*Page(s)*
1. Not known				
2. Heterosexual sex				
3. Homosexual sex				
4. Intravenous drug use				
5. Blood/blood products				
6. Vertical transmission				
7. Multiple risk factors				
8. Other				

WHAT ARE THE EXPLICIT FEARS OF PROTAGONISTS CONCERNING HIV/AIDS?

Book Title: ______________________ Coder Name: ______________

Does the Protagonist Feel at Risk?	*Relevant Content*	*Page(s)*
1. Not sure		
2. Not indicated		
3. No		
4. Yes, fear for self		
5. Yes, fear for other(s)		

ARE THERE INDICATIONS THAT DISEASE CAN BE CONTROLLED?

Book Title: ______________________ Coder Name: ______________

Indication That Disease Can Be Controlled	*Relevant Content*	*Page(s)*

WHAT IS THE FATE OF HIV/AIDS CHARACTERS IN THESE STORIES?

Book Title: ______________________________ Coder Name: ________________

Do They Die?	*Relevant Content*	*Page(s)*
1. Text doesn't say		
2. Dies		
3. Dying or death imminent		
4. Lives		
5. Other outcome		

Index

About the Authors

Melissa Gross is a professor in the School of Library and Information Science at Florida State University. Her research specialty is information seeking behavior. Current projects include investigations into the information literacy needs of undergraduates and the HIV/AIDS content of materials developed for a young adult audience. Gross's most recent books are *Studying Children's Questions: Imposed and Self-Generated Information Seeking at School*, published by Scarecrow Press in 2006, and *Dynamic Youth Services through Outcome Based Planning and Evaluation*, coauthored with Eliza Dresang and Leslie Holt, published by ALA Publications in 2006.

Annette Y. Goldsmith is a lecturer at the University of Washington Information School and founding editor of *The Looking Glass* (www.lib.latrobe.edu.au/ojs/index.php/tlg/index). Her area of expertise is international children's literature. Goldsmith has chaired the Mildred L. Batchelder Award Committee, which recognizes the publisher of the most outstanding children's book translation published in the United States, and has been a member of the United States Board on Books for Young People Outstanding International Books Committee.

Debi Carruth is a doctoral candidate at the Florida State University College of Communication and Information. Her primary research examines the information behaviors of gifted youth in everyday life, particularly related to their hobby pursuits.

LaVergne, TN USA
22 September 2010
198117LV00001B/2/P